Chef Erin's
GLUTEN-FREE
Cookbook

500+ GLUTEN-FREE RECIPES FOR BEGINNER
AND EXPERIENCED HOME COOKS

Recipes for multiple dietary lifestyles, including Traditional Comfort Food,
Dairy-Free, Low-Carb, Mediterranean, Plant-Based, Vegan, and Vegetarian

Erin K. Courtney

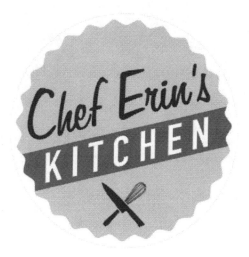

www.cheferinskitchen.com

Chef Erin's Gluten-Free Cookbook

ISBN: 979-8-853172-66-1

The information provided in this book should not be used for diagnosing or treating a health problem or disease, and those seeking personal medical advice should consult with a licensed physician. Always seek the advice of your doctor or other qualified health provider regarding a medical condition. The author and publisher shall have neither liability nor responsibility to anyone with respect to any loss or damage caused, or alleged to be caused, directly or indirectly by the information provided in this book.

This book is available at www.amazon.com

Other Books Written by Erin K. Courtney

Freezer Pleasers
Over 150 delicious make-ahead recipes to keep your freezer stocked
for all meals and occasions!

What's for Dinner?
Over 115 quick and easy recipes for breakfast and brunch, salads & sandwiches, entrees
(chicken, beef, pork, & vegetarian), side dishes, and desserts!

All I Want Is Cheesecake
Over 75 recipes of mouth-watering New York style cheesecakes
that are sure to satisfy every sweet tooth craving!

Party Time!
Over 200 easy party food recipes! Includes recipes for:
hot appetizers, cold appetizers, beverages (both kid-friendly and adult),
self-serve desserts and crowd-pleasing desserts!

101 Reasons to Run
This cute, funny, and motivational book gives you 101 reasons to get going for a run so
you'll have no reason not to! This is a perfect gift for runners, or anyone who can enjoy a
good laugh at these educational and ridiculous reasons to go for a run.

101 Reasons to Drink Coffee
Not like you need a reason to drink coffee, but just in case you do, here are 101 logical
and snarky reasons to indulge in the greatest beverage known to mankind.

Intermittent Fasting Journal
An introduction that eases you into some basic information about Intermittent Fasting,
along with health benefits, success stories, motivational quotes, and daily journal entries
to get you started on your Fasting Path!

Recipes I Stole
This blank recipe journal is the perfect way to gather all the recipes you have stolen from
other people. It's for a collection of recipes that were so delicious they were practically
begged to be stolen and made their way into your own personal recipe library.

...AND MANY MORE!!!

Available at www.amazon.com

About the Author

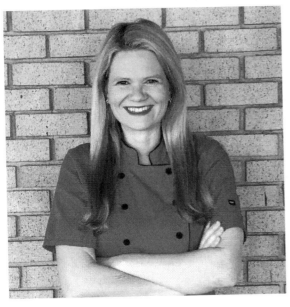

Erin K. Courtney did not learn how to cook growing up. Her parents worked many hours running a business and trying to raise three crazy kids, so there was very little time to cook anything other than something that came out of a box. She was in her early thirties before she ever baked a cake; that's when a pastry class at her local community college opened the floodgates. Erin started baking and decorating cakes several times a week, sending the finished products to work with her husband and sister-in-law. After a few more classes, she started experimenting with different dessert items. Friends flocked to her for birthday confections, and the dessert table at family gatherings became quite elaborate.

Two years after Erin's first cake-decorating class, she started a one-year culinary program at the University of South Carolina. Now able to cook impressive homemade meals, Erin still found herself searching for simplicity. She continued to obsessively experiment with different recipes, looking for ways to streamline challenging ones and incorporate ingredients that were easy to find at local grocery stores.

Now, like the teacher whose helpful advice drew her into the world of baking, Erin wants to share her discoveries with novice chefs in her cookbooks. From party menus to desserts to multi-course feasts to freezer meals and healthier options, Erin hopes her research and experience will help readers of every skill level make easy, tasty, kid-friendly food.

She has been the featured chef on HTC's Inside Out TV show based in Myrtle Beach, along with a live interview on WPDE Carolina and Company Live, and has been featured in the Food and Beverage section of The Sun News. Erin hosts live demonstration dinner parties in her home, offering hands-on instructions for her party guests. She stuffs their bellies with multiple recipes along with answering any questions her guests have. She also teaches instructional cooking demonstrations at local venues in her community.

Erin is married to the greatest guy on the planet, they have two ridiculously cute kids and reside in South Carolina. After finishing certification programs through the Institute of Integrative Nutrition and the Academy of Culinary Nutrition, she hopes to help shed some light for other people through their own personal health journeys.

Chef Erin's Gluten-Free Cookbook

In 2017, I was diagnosed with three different digestive disorders (Irritable Bowel Syndrome, Gastritis, and Small Intestinal Bacterial Overgrowth) on top of an autoimmune disease. The medications I was given weren't helping my health issues at all, and I felt incredibly lost and hopeless. Desperate for improvement, I removed gluten from my diet as an experiment after doing some research. In less than one week, my Psoriasis cleared up completely, along with my digestive issues that drastically improved. Curious about what would happen, I threw gluten back into my body and the problems returned with a vengeance within 24 hours. Since I was working in the restaurant industry as a pastry chef, my heart sank when I realized that changing my diet was crucial if I wanted to stop feeling sick all the time. The fire that I had as a passion for cooking started to diminish when such a monumental ingredient was being eliminated from most of the recipes I had already developed. I was devastated.

When I pulled out my culinary school textbook and started thumbing through dishes for ideas, it reminded me how many real ingredients were used in most of these recipes; meaning many of them were already naturally gluten-free without having to make any adjustments. It dawned on me how a massive collection of recipes was about to spiral out of control, and a smile spread across my face that resembled the Grinch right before he stole Christmas. That smile returned many times as I was compiling all these recipes and couldn't wait to make them...*ALL* of them. My spark had re-ignited.

After publishing my first four traditional cookbooks that weren't gluten-free, many friends and family started asking me for gluten-free recipes since they were experiencing health issues of their own. Although several recipes from my first books were technically gluten-free, people were looking for a collection of recipes that fell into that category of being *only* gluten-free; and they wanted more. So, this book was born.

This book is a collection of recipes from my previous books that have been transformed into gluten-free, in addition to many other recipes that I converted into being gluten-free or discovered through a massive amount of research online and through multiple cookbooks. Out of my entire cookbook library, this is the book I use the most.

My main goal with writing this book is to provide you with as many recipes as possible so you can cook satisfying meals at home without having to sacrifice taste. I also hope you can start tricking people into eating healthier items the way I have, so maybe we can even start a Sneaky Chef Club. I hope this book can help you enjoy cooking again the way it has done for myself, family, and friends. Let's eat, I'm hungry.

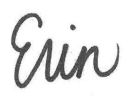

Kitchen
CONVERSIONS

1 GALLON
4 QUARTS
8 PINTS
16 CUPS
128 OUNCES
3.8 LITERS

1 QUART
2 PINTS
4 CUPS
32 OUNCES
950 ML

1 PINT
2 CUPS
16 OUNCES
480 ML

1 CUP
16 TBSP
1/2 PINT
8 OUNCES
240 ML

1/4 CUP
4 TBSP
12 TSP
2 OUNCES
60 ML

1 TBSP
3 TSP
1/2 OUNCE
15 ML

Contents

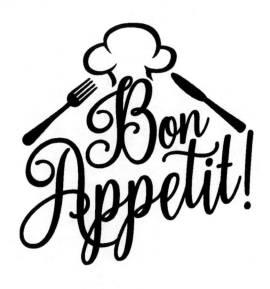

Introduction

What is Gluten?
Other than being the devil for certain people, gluten is a protein found in many grains, including wheat, barley, and rye. It is composed of two smaller proteins (gliadin and glutenin) that give wheat-based dough its elasticity and sticky consistency. It is commonly found in traditional breads, pastas, pastries, and many other foods made with wheat, barley, or rye flour. It's also a sneaky little devil that is used in many other products that you wouldn't think, which is why checking labels is so important.

Gluten Sensitivity
Also known as non-celiac gluten sensitivity, a condition when a person experiences symptoms after consuming gluten-containing foods but does not have Celiac Disease or a wheat allergy. Symptoms can include digestive issues such as bloating, diarrhea, abdominal pain, along with fatigue, brain fog and joint pain. Although the exact cause is not well understood, it is believed to be related to an immune system response to gluten.

Gluten Intolerance
This is more of a broad term that can refer to several different conditions in which a person has difficulty digesting gluten. It can include Celiac Disease, Non-Celiac Gluten Sensitivity, Irritable Bowel Syndrome and Inflammatory Bowel Disease. The symptoms vary widely and depend on the specific condition, but can include digestive issues, fatigue, join pain, along with many other issues.

Gluten Allergy
Also known as Wheat Allergy, is an immune system response to wheat proteins, including gluten and is an IgE-medicated allergic reaction. When a person with a wheat allergy consumes wheat or gluten, the immune system releases histamines that can cause symptoms such as hives, itching, swelling, difficulty breathing, or even anaphylaxis. Gluten Sensitivity and Intolerance can be managed through dietary changes and lifestyle modifications, but a Wheat Allergy requires strict avoidance of wheat and gluten-containing foods and products. It is definitely the devil in this case.

Celiac Disease
Celiac Disease is a genetic autoimmune disorder where the immune system reacts abnormally to gluten. When someone with Celiac consumes gluten, their immune system attacks the lining of the small intestine, causing damage to the villi (small finger-like projections that absorb nutrients from food). Damage to the villi can lead to malabsorption of nutrients and a wide range of symptoms, including abdominal pain, bloating, diarrhea, constipation, weight loss, fatigue, anemia, join pain, and skin rashes.

This is a chronic condition with no cure, but it can be managed through a gluten-free lifestyle by avoiding all sources of gluten. If left untreated, it can lead to serious health complications, such as malnutrition, osteoporosis, and increased risk of certain cancers.

If you think you may have Celiac Disease, it may be best to get a blood test done before removing gluten for an accurate test result. Although the number of people diagnosed with Celiac Disease is still very low compared to the entire population, the number is on the rise. It's genetic, so if a family member has Celiac Disease or other gluten sensitivity, there's an increased possibility that other family members can have it as well.

Why Eliminate Gluten?
Eliminating gluten from your diet is necessary if you have Celiac Disease or other listed issues above to reduce symptoms and improve your overall health.

Is it GLUTEN or GLYPHOSATE?
My family physician is really into nutrition, but practices at a place where not many people share his similar passion. Knowing this about him, I always bring up nutrition at my appointments and he is more than delighted to talk about it. The problem is that his level of knowledge and understanding with his medical background has my head spinning in circles when he unloads new information on me all at once, but I learn something new from every single appointment. If I really want to get him fired up and talk about lifestyle, all I must mention is Intermittent Fasting. He is a *huge* fan.

One day while I was chatting with him about gluten, he brought up Glyphosate and how it's used in our country on wheat products. "Before you eliminate gluten completely, you might want to experiment with organic flour and other products containing gluten to see if your system tolerates those a little better. Your body could be reacting to the chemicals instead of the gluten itself." I sat there and stared at him, wondering if he could see the lightbulb appear above my head. "Is that why I keep hearing why the United States is basically the only country in the world where people have so many issues with gluten, is because of the chemicals used on our food?" He smiled and nodded, then recommended reading *Metabolical* by Robert H. Lustig, MD. That book was extremely informative.

Intermittent Fasting for Digestive Issues
Intermittent Fasting (IF) is an eating pattern that alternates periods of fasting and eating. IF may be beneficial for people with digestive issues because it gives the digestive system a break in order to rest and repair. When we eat, our digestive system works very hard to break down and absorb nutrients from food. By fasting for a period of time, it helps reduce inflammation and improve gut health. It can also help regulate the gut microbiome, which is the collection of microorganisms that live in our gut and play a critical role in digestion and overall health (especially since 70% of the immune system resides in the gut). IF can increase the diversity of the gut microbiome and promote the growth of beneficial bacteria, which can help alleviate digestive symptoms.

For me personally, daily Intermittent Fasting (13-16 hours) has helped heal my gut tremendously and I plan to continue this lifestyle for the rest of my life. I have written a book for beginners looking to experiment with IF, called *Intermittent Fasting Journal: an Introduction to Intermittent Fasting and One-Year Journal*. If you're looking for more information on IF, check out *Fast. Feast. Repeat.* by Gin Stephens, along with her Intermittent Fasting Podcast. I was a guest on her IF Stories Podcast, episode #331 if you would like to listen to my goofy voice explain in depth my personal journey.

Is it a GLUTEN Issue or a FODMAP Issue?
It can be challenging to figure out if you're having an issue with gluten or FODMAPs (Fermentable Oligosaccharides, Disaccharides, Monosaccharides, and Polyols) since the symptoms of these two conditions can overlap.

FODMAPs are a group of short-chain carbohydrates that are poorly absorbed in the small intestine and can ferment in the large intestine, leading to symptoms such as bloating, gas, and abdominal pain. FODMAPs are found in wheat, rye, barley, along with certain fruits, vegetables, and dairy products. If you think you may have an issue with FODMAPs, a healthcare professional, registered dietitian or nutritionist should be able to help you figure out what's best for you.

ALWAYS, ALWAYS, ALWAYS CHECK LABELS!!!
Although I have researched and tested so many recipes, there are some brands that are certified gluten-free while others are not. For instance, Jell-O® pudding. Jell-O® instant pudding mix that I have used in many recipes over the years IS certified gluten-free, while the generic version of the same pudding mix is NOT certified gluten-free and isn't safe for someone with Celiac Disease or a severe allergy. Pudding mix is just one example of all the products available, so be sure to triple-check the labels depending on your level of sensitivity, intolerance, or allergy. This is in reference to ALL packaged items, including sauces, soups, seasonings, and any other mixes. Gluten is in many other products, such as supplements, medications, beauty products, and even toothpaste.

Gluten-Free App
Checking ingredients and labels for the Certified Gluten-Free label can get overwhelming when you first start out, which is why having the app on your phone is incredibly helpful. It scans the bar code and lets you know the status of a product, whether it's Certified Gluten-Free, No Gluten Containing Ingredients, or Contains Gluten. This is a wonderful app to have on your phone while grocery shopping, and I have been known to whip out my phone to scan a barcode on more occasions than I can remember, but it's a wonderful tool to have on hand. If you hear me cry out, "Yes!" after scanning an item at the store, this is probably the reason for it.

Product Availability
Always check product availability based on your location. Finding ingredients can be simple or challenging depending on where you live. All the recipes in this book are based on ingredients that can be found in the Southeastern United States. If you live somewhere else and a recipe calls for a specific ingredient you can't get your hands on, an internet search is a great way to find substitutions to use in its place, whether you need to order online, find in a different store, or improvise with substitutions.

Dairy-Free Conversions
Many recipes can be converted to dairy-free simply by replacing regular butter with plant butter, and regular milk with non-dairy milk. There are many options for dairy-free milk, whether it's oat, almond, rice, cashew, coconut, etc. Some milks have a thicker consistency than others, but many of them can be used in recipes that call for regular milk. If you have nut allergies, oat or rice milk for the win!

Check out the Specialty Diet Recipe Index on page 228!
This section categorizes recipes based on different diets, so you can narrow down specific recipes for different preferences. You can use different colors of sticky notes to tag types of recipes for easy organization. It's also helpful if you have family or friends coming over for dinner with dietary restrictions, and it gives you more options to be a star chef who saved the day by making incredible food for everyone. You're welcome.

What kind of gluten-free all-purpose flour to use in recipes?
Depending on the recipe, you can use a traditional all-purpose gluten-free flour blend that is available in many grocery stores or make your own blend to keep on hand.

Flours that contain xanthan gum are not the best choice for using in sauces, because it gives the sauce a gummy texture.
For example, Cup4Cup®, Better Batter®, and Bob's Red Mill® brands do contain xanthan gum, whereas King Arthur® flour does NOT contain xanthan gum. This is a great storebought flour to use for making a roux (butter + flour) as a thickening agent for sauces. Please trust me on this, I learned the hard way while making an Alfredo sauce that ended up having a gummy texture. It did not affect the taste, but it did affect the texture. ***Look for the no XG in the list of ingredients!***

Using UNsalted Butter in Recipes
This was an early question I asked in culinary school, and it makes so much sense. When cooking you can always ADD extra seasonings if you need it, but you can't take it away. By using unsalted butter, you can determine how salty or unsalty your recipe comes out. Too much salt in a meal can lead to making faces like the first time a baby sucks on a lemon. It's entertaining to everyone else watching, but not so much for the victim.

What kind of bread to use?
This can get tricky, because it's hard to find storebought gluten-free bread that is as delicious as traditional bread. This is trial-and-error, so you can experiment with different brands to see which ones you like the best. I typically buy my gluten-free bread from the frozen section and thaw it out as needed. If you make your own gluten-free bread, wrapping it in plastic wrap and freezing it will help preserve freshness.

What kind of pasta to use?
There are a ton of options these days for using gluten-free pasta, and one of the best things about these new products is that most people don't even realize it's gluten-free. When I switched our Spaghetti Night to gluten-free, I used the Ronzoni® brand of thin spaghetti. Did anyone in my family notice? They did not. Unfortunately, my poker face is terrible, and my husband started questioning why I had a smirk on my face after asking everyone if they enjoyed their dinner. Busted and proud.

Brown rice and chickpea pasta is wonderful for serving immediately but doesn't reheat or bake well. It takes a longer to cook but is very filling. Ronzoni® brand pasta is my personal favorite to use when tricking people into eating gluten-free without even realizing it. There are other blends to choose from as well using different flours, so you can experiment with different brands to see which works best for you and your family.

Cooked Bacon Bits vs. Cooking Real Bacon
Many recipes in this book call for Cooked Bacon Bits for one reason and one reason only: convenience. Well, and a little bit of laziness on my end, especially since I love shortcuts. If you would prefer to cook your own bacon and reserve the fat for incredible flavor, please feel free to do so. If you decide to do this, here is the conversion:
1 slice bacon = 1 tablespoon real bacon bits

Certified Gluten-Free vs. Does Not Have Gluten Containing Ingredients
You may notice some items are labeled differently when you start looking for gluten-free items. Certified Gluten-Free means that the product is made in a gluten-free facility so there is no chance of cross-contamination. If it's labeled Does Not Have Gluten Containing Ingredients, that just means the ingredients alone do not contain gluten, but it's not made in a dedicated gluten-free facility and there *is* a possibility of cross-contamination. This is an important difference if you have Celiac Disease or an allergy.

Using Cooked Chicken in Recipes
*Buy raw chicken and cook it yourself, dividing it into portions and freezing it for later.
*Buy a cooked rotisserie chicken and separate the meat from the bones. This gives you a variety of meat from the different parts of the chicken without having to cook it yourself.
*Buy the pre-cooked chicken in bags, which only needs to be reheated.
*Buy cooked chicken in cans, drain and measure when preparing in recipes.

Salt and Pepper To Taste
You'll notice that some recipes call for specific amounts of salt and pepper, whereas others call for salt and pepper to taste. This is because some recipes require a certain amount, when others are your call on how salty and peppery you like your food. When in doubt, always consult the professionals...Salt 'n Pepa.

Exercise for Digestive Discomfort
Fun Fact: regular exercise can help reduce constipation, inflammation, stress, and promote a healthy gut microbiome diversity. Even a daily walk can make a significant positive difference in overall health. Core workouts strengthen the abdomen, improving circulation that can help improve digestion and nutrient absorption. Strong core muscles also help move waste through the system more efficiently, promoting bowel regularity and reducing constipation. It can be a mood killer to stay backed up.

Personally, yoga provides immediate relief when I suffer from digestive discomfort. Certain yoga postures can help to stimulate the digestive system and improve circulation to the abdomen, which can help alleviate discomfort. It also promotes the relaxation response in the body, which can help improve digestion. Just be prepared for the possibility of a little bit of gas being released in the process, which is why I do yoga in the comfort of my own home. Don't say I didn't warn you.

This is an American Cookbook, so most measurements are in cups and teaspoons, and temperatures are in Fahrenheit. Please see kitchen chart on page 6 for measurement conversions.

Beginner 🥄   Intermediate 🥄🥄   Experienced 🥄🥄🥄

Each recipe will be labeled with the number of whisks to determine if it's at a beginner, intermediate, or experienced level of cooking. Many of the recipes in this book fall under the first two categories, but as your kitchen skills improve or you have more time for preparation and cooking, your recipe options increase and you become a culinary ninja!

🥄 **Beginner Level:** if you're just starting out with cooking or are looking to save time with something quick and easy involving less time and ingredients.

🥄🥄 **Intermediate Level:** middle of the road recipes that may require a little more prep, time, or ingredients than beginner level but are not too challenging.

🥄🥄🥄 **Experienced Level:** you're a seasoned home cook or chef, have plenty of time, and have no problem dirtying your kitchen for a fantastic meal fit for a King and Queen.

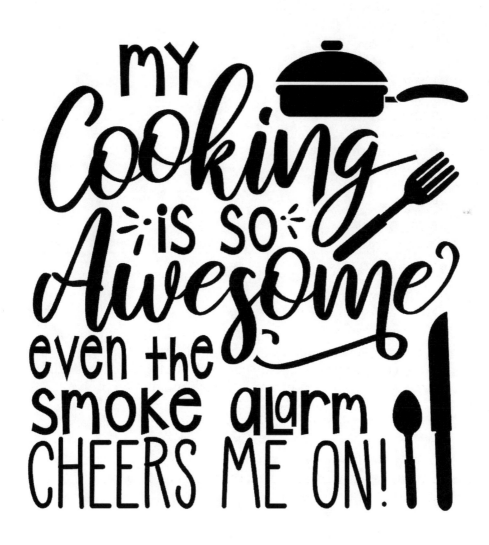

Hot & Cold Appetizers

Asian Lettuce Wraps 🍴 *(6-8 servings)*

1 lb. ground chicken
1 tbsp. peanut oil
½ cup diced onion
1 cup diced bell pepper (green or red)
8 oz. can water chestnuts, drained and minced
6 tbsp. gluten-free soy sauce

½ teaspoon garlic powder
1 tbsp. rice wine vinegar
2 tsp. chili sauce
16 Boston Bibb lettuce leaves
1 bunch green onions, minced

Rinse and pat dry lettuce leaves, set aside. Heat oil in skillet on medium/high heat, add ground chicken and cook completely. Drain meat, return to skillet and add onion and peppers, cook until soft. Add water chestnuts and stir. Add soy sauce, rice wine vinegar, chili sauce, and garlic powder. Stir until chicken and vegetables are evenly coated. Serve in lettuce leaves and garnish with green onions.

Bacon Wrapped Asparagus 🍴 *(6-8 servings)*

24 stalks asparagus, trimmed
12 slices bacon

½ tbsp. olive oil
½ tsp. black pepper

Preheat oven to 400 degrees, line a baking sheet with foil or parchment paper. Place the asparagus in a large mixing bowl, drizzle with olive oil, sprinkle with pepper and toss to coat. Slice the bacon lengthwise to make thin strips. Tightly wrap each slice of bacon around each piece of asparagus, place seam side down on baking sheet. Place sheet in oven and bake for 15-20 minutes, until bacon is crispy, and asparagus is tender.

Bacon Wrapped Hot Dog Bites 🍴 *(6-8 servings)*

12 slices bacon, cut in half
6 gluten-free hot dogs, cut into 4 pieces

¼ cup light brown sugar
¼ cup butter, melted

Preheat oven to 400 degrees, press foil into and up edges of cookie sheet. Wrap 1 bacon piece around each hot dog piece, stick a toothpick through (this keeps the bacon and hot dog piece together), place seam-side down on foil. In a small mixing bowl, whisk together brown sugar and melted butter until dissolved, drizzle on top of hot dogs. Bake a total of 22-24 minutes, or until bacon is crisp and golden brown, flipping once after 12 minutes. Serve warm.

Bacon Wrapped Jalapeno Poppers *(6-8 servings)*

12 jalapeno peppers
8 oz. cream cheese, softened
1 cup grated pepper jack cheese

½ tsp. onion powder
12 slices bacon

Preheat oven to 400 degrees, line a sheet pan with foil or parchment paper. Cut the jalapenos in half lengthwise, scoop out seeds and ribs with a spoon. In a medium size mixing bowl, combine cream cheese, pepper jack cheese, onion powder, and beat with electric mixer until well combined. Fill each half of jalapeno peppers with cheese mixture. Cut each slice of bacon in half, wrap around each pepper and secure with a toothpick. Place peppers on baking sheet and bake for 20-25 minutes, until bacon is crispy and peppers are tender.

Bacon Wrapped Shrimp *(6-8 servings)*

16 large shrimp, peeled and deveined (with tails)
8 slices bacon, cut in half crosswise

2 tbsp. butter, melted
1 tsp. chili powder

Preheat oven to 425 degrees, line a sheet pan with foil or parchment paper. In a small bowl, whisk together melted butter and chili powder. Toss with shrimp in a medium size mixing bowl, until shrimp are evenly coated. Wrap each shrimp with a piece of bacon, secure with a toothpick. Place shrimp on pan, bake for about 15 minutes or until bacon is crispy and shrimp is cooked.

Pro-Tip: when it comes to shrimp tails in recipes, most of the time this is a preference. For me personally, I prefer no tails simply because that means I have to remove the tails before eating the shrimp. Anything to slow down the process when it's actually time to eat just gets in the way, but that's just me. I know a lot of people who prefer to have shrimp with the tails. You do you, boo.

BBQ Chicken Wings *(6-8 servings)*

1 (about 2 ½ lbs.) bag frozen chicken wingettes
1 (12 oz.) bottle gluten-free BBQ sauce

½ cup ranch dressing
¼ cup light brown sugar

Place frozen chicken in slow cooker and turn setting to low. In a small mixing bowl, whisk together BBQ sauce, ranch and brown sugar. Whisk until mixed well; pour over chicken. Cover and cook on low for 3-4 hours, stirring chicken around in sauce after 1-2 hours. Make sure chicken wings reach internal temp of 165 degrees before serving.

Hot Chicken Wings ⅋ *(6-8 servings)*

1 (about 2 ½ lbs.) bag frozen chicken wingettes ½ cup unsalted butter
1 (12 oz.) bottle hot sauce

Place frozen chicken in slow cooker and turn setting to low. Combine hot sauce and butter in a small saucepan. Cook on low/medium heat until butter has melted, pour over chicken in slow cooker. Cover and cook on low for 3-4 hours, stirring chicken around in sauce after 1-2 hours. Make sure chicken wings reach internal temp of 165 degrees.

Honey Mustard Chicken Wings ⅋ *(6-8 servings)*

1 (about 2 ½ lbs.) bag frozen chicken wingettes   ¾ cup Dijon mustard
¾ cup honey   ¼ cup unsalted butter, melted

Place frozen chicken wings in slow cooker, turn to low setting. In a small mixing bowl, whisk together honey, mustard, and melted butter until smooth, pour over chicken. Cover and cook on low for 3-4 hours, stirring chicken around in sauce after 1-2 hours. Make sure chicken wings reach internal temp of 165 degrees.

Buffalo Cheesy Chicken Dip ⅋ *(10-12 servings)*

1 (12.5 oz.) can chunk white chicken, drained   ¾ cup buffalo wing sauce
1 (8 oz.) package cream cheese, softened   1 cup grated Monterey jack cheese
¾ cup ranch dressing   1 cup grated sharp cheddar cheese

Combine all ingredients in medium mixing bowl, beat at medium speed with electric mixer until well blended. Spoon mixture into 1 ½ quart slow cooker, cook on low until completely melted, 2-4 hours, stirring occasionally. Switch setting to warm when mixture is melted to prevent burning. Serve warm with tortilla chips.

Black Bean and Corn Salsa ⅋ *(14-16 servings)*

15.5 oz. jar salsa   1 cup frozen corn, thawed
15 oz. can black beans, rinsed and drained   1 cup diced onion

Combine all ingredients in mixing bowl, gently stir and combine well. Serve with tortilla chips. Store in airtight container in refrigerator for up to 7 days.

Buffalo Turkey Meatballs *(10-12 servings)*

30 oz. bag gluten-free frozen turkey meatballs
16 oz. bottle Buffalo wing sauce

1 cup ranch dressing
½ cup light brown sugar

Coat a 4-quart slow cooker with cooking spray, lay meatballs inside. In a small mixing bowl, whisk together wing sauce, ranch dressing, and light brown sugar. Pour on top of meatballs, cook on low for 2 hours until hot. Turn setting to warm and serve.

Charcuterie Board *(6-8 servings)*

8 oz. cured meat (prosciutto, salami)
8 oz. soft cheese (brie, goat cheese)
8 oz. hard cheese (gruyere, cheddar, gouda)
8 oz. gluten-free crackers

¼ cup jam
½ cup mixed nuts
2 cups grapes

Arrange meats in the center of a charcuterie board (or large cutting board). Cut cheeses into small cubes. Surround meats with cheeses and crackers. Spoon jam, mixed nuts, and grapes into their own small bowls and place on board for serving.

Cheddar Bacon Dip *(12-14 servings)*

1 cup milk
8 oz. sour cream
8 oz. cream cheese, softened

3 cups grated cheddar cheese, divided
0.4 oz. packet ranch dressing mix
½ cup real bacon bits

Preheat oven to 350 degrees. In a medium sized mixing bowl, combine all ingredients, reserving 1 cup grated cheddar cheese. Beat at medium speed with electric mixer until mixture is well combined. Spoon into a 9-inch round pie dish or 8x8 inch square baking dish. Sprinkle with reserved 1 cup cheddar. Bake for 20-25 minutes, or until cheeses are melted and bubbling. Serve warm with gluten-free crackers or tortilla chips.

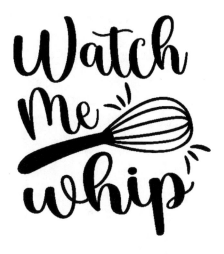

Cheddar Cheese Ball *(16-20 servings)*

2 (8 oz.) packages cream cheese, softened
2 green onions, diced
1 tsp. gluten-free Worcestershire sauce
½ tsp. garlic powder

1 tsp. Italian seasoning
2 cups freshly grated sharp cheddar
½ cup pecans, finely chopped

Place softened cream cheese, onions, Worcestershire, and seasonings in a medium size mixing bowl. Beat with electric mixer until smooth. Add cheddar cheese, beat again until well combined. Place a large piece of plastic wrap on a work surface. Spoon mixture out of bowl and onto the plastic wrap. Completely wrap the cheese ball in the plastic wrap, smoothing and shaping as you wrap it up into a ball. Set in refrigerator for at least 2 hours before serving. Remove from fridge about an hour before serving to let cheese ball soften slightly, gently press in chopped pecans. Store leftovers in airtight container in refrigerator for up to 5 days.

Cheese Fries *(6-8 servings)*

1 (20 oz.) bag frozen French fries
1 cup milk

4 cups grated sharp cheddar cheese
½ cup real bacon bits

Cook fries according to package directions (baking or frying). While fries are cooking, prepare the cheese sauce. In a medium saucepan, heat milk on medium heat until hot. Add cheese, continue to whisk as cheese melts. When fries are done cooking, place in a 9x13 inch baking dish or a serving platter. Pour cheese sauce over fries and top with bacon bits. Serve warm.

Cheesy Bean Dip *(16-18 servings)*

1 (20 oz.) can refried pinto beans
8 oz. cream cheese, softened

8 oz. sour cream
2 cups grated sharp cheddar cheese

In a medium mixing bowl, combine all ingredients. Beat with electric mixer at medium speed for about 2 minutes or until mixture is well-combined. Spoon into a 1 ½ quart slow cooker, turn to low setting, and cook for 2-3 hours or until cheese is melted and mixture is hot. Turn knob to warm setting, serve with tortilla chips.

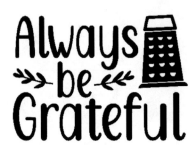

Cheesy Sausage Balls ĭ *(40 sausage balls)*

1 lb. ground pork sausage   1 lb. grated sharp cheddar cheese
2 cups gluten-free baking mix (like Bisquick®)

Preheat oven to 400 degrees. Combine all ingredients in a medium size mixing bowl and mix well with hands until thoroughly combined. Roll into 1-inch balls, place on cookie sheet, and bake for 12-15 minutes or until golden brown and sausage is cooked through. These can be prepared ahead of time and frozen; thaw completely in refrigerator and cook as above or increase baking time to 20-22 minutes.

Chicken Bites ĭ *(6-8 servings)*

24 oz. bag gluten-free frozen boneless chicken nuggets/bites
1 cup gluten-free BBQ sauce

Cook chicken according to package directions. When chicken bites are done baking, toss together in a medium size mixing bowl with BBQ sauce until evenly coated, serve with toothpicks. **Change up the sauce for a variety of flavors!** You can use hot sauce, ranch dressing, honey mustard, etc.

Chicken Cheese Ball ĭ *(16-20 servings)*

2 (8 oz.) packages cream cheese, softened   5 oz. can cooked chicken
1 (0.4 oz.) packet ranch dressing

In a medium mixing bowl, combine all ingredients. Using an electric mixer, beat at medium speed for about 2 minutes until all ingredients are well-blended. Place a large piece of plastic wrap on a work surface. Spoon mixture out of bowl and onto the plastic wrap. Completely wrap the cheese ball in the plastic wrap, smoothing and shaping as you wrap it up into a ball. Set in refrigerator for at least 2 hours before serving. Remove from fridge about an hour before serving to let cheese ball soften slightly, serve with gluten-free crackers. Store leftovers in airtight container in refrigerator for up to 5 days.

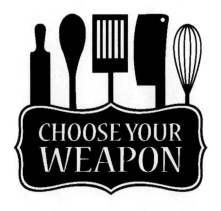

CHOOSE YOUR WEAPON

Chicken Quesadillas *(4 servings)*

4 gluten-free tortillas
4 oz. cooked chicken, diced
4 oz. grated sharp cheddar cheese

4 oz. grated pepper jack cheese
taco seasoning

Heat an electric skillet to 300 degrees or a non-stick pan on medium heat on the stove. Spray the pan with cooking spray, then place a tortilla on top. Sprinkle about 1 oz. of each cheese on the tortilla, followed by ½ teaspoon seasoning. Sprinkle 1 oz. chicken on one side of the tortilla (since you'll be folding it over), cook for about two minutes. Using a pair of tongs, slightly pull up the side with no chicken to check the bottom. When the bottom is light golden, fold it over on top of the other half. Continue to cook for about 1 minute, just until the cheese is melted. You can flip the quesadilla over, making sure each side is cooked evenly and cheeses are melted. Transfer finished quesadilla to a plate to cool slightly before slicing with a pizza cutter. Serve with Quesadilla Sauce (page 34) on the side for dipping, or drizzle on top.

Chili Cheese Tots *(6-8 servings)*

32 oz. bag frozen tater tots
3 cups grated sharp cheddar cheese

15 oz. can gluten-free chili
1 cup milk

Cook tater tots according to package directions. In a medium sauce pan, combine chili, milk, and cheese, cook on medium heat until hot and cheese is melted. Spoon on top of tater tots and serve warm.

Chocolate Cheese Ball *(8-12 servings)*

8 oz. cream cheese, softened
¼ cup butter, softened
1 cup confectioners sugar

1 tsp. vanilla extract
¼ cup unsweetened cocoa
½ cup mini chocolate chips

In a medium size mixing bowl, combine cream cheese and butter. Beat with electric mixer at medium speed until creamy. Add powdered sugar, vanilla, and cocoa powder. Continue beating at medium speed until all ingredients are well-blended and creamy. Place a piece of plastic wrap on a clean counter, spoon cheese ball on top of plastic wrap. Fully wrap the cheese ball, shaping into a smooth ball. Store in refrigerator for at least 2 hour before serving. Remove from refrigerator at least 30 minutes before serving to let cheese ball soften for easier spreading, roll in mini chocolate chips. Serve with gluten-free graham crackers, cookies, and/or pretzels.

Chocolate Covered Stuffed Strawberries ♔ *(10-12 servings)*

1 lb. fresh strawberries
8 oz. cream cheese, softened
1/3 cup confectioners sugar

1 tsp. vanilla extract
½ pound dark chocolate (wafers or chips)

Rinse strawberries in cold water, pat dry with paper towels. Cut off the stem of each strawberry, creating a flat top, set aside. Take a paring knife and hollow out a small section for the filling. In a small mixing bowl, combine cream cheese, powdered sugar and vanilla. Beat with electric mixer at medium speed until mixture is creamy. Spoon mixture into a pastry bag or freezer bag and cut off the tip. Squeeze mixture into the hollow cavity of each strawberry. Once strawberries are filled with cheesecake mixture, set aside. Melt chocolate in microwave safe dish in microwave in 15-20 second intervals, stirring in between each interval until melted and smooth. Pick up each strawberry at the top (where the stuffing is coming out), dip the bottom in melted chocolate, and place on a wax paper-lined cookie sheet. After all strawberries have been dipped, place cookie sheet in refrigerator for at least 10 minutes for chocolate to harden. Remove from cookie sheet and serve immediately, or store in refrigerator until ready to serve.

Pro-Tip: strawberries need to be completely dry before dipping in chocolate, or the chocolate won't stick!

Cocktail Weenies ♔ *(80 weenies)*

2 (14 oz.) packs gluten-free lil' smokies
12 oz. grape jelly

12 oz. bottle chili sauce
½ cup light brown sugar

In small saucepan, combine chili sauce, jelly, and sugar. Cook on medium heat until jelly melts and mixture is smooth. Place sausage links in slow cooker, pour mixture on top, and cook on low for 2-3 hours. Turn setting to warm and serve.

Cookie Dough Dip ♔ *(8-12 servings)*

8 oz. cream cheese, softened
½ cup unsalted butter, softened
½ cup confectioners sugar

¼ cup light brown sugar
1 tsp. vanilla
1 cup mini chocolate chips

In a medium size mixing bowl, combine cream cheese and butter. Beat with electric mixer at medium speed until creamy. Add both sugars and vanilla. Continue beating at medium speed until all ingredients are well-blended and creamy. Stir in mini chocolate chips. Spoon into a small serving bowl, cover with plastic wrap and store in refrigerator for at least 2 hours before serving. Remove from refrigerator at least 30 minutes before serving to let it soften. Serve with gluten-free graham crackers, cookies, and/or pretzels.

Creamy Corn Dip *(14-16 servings)*

1 cup mayonnaise
½ tsp. salt
1 tsp. onion powder
1 cup grated Monterey jack cheese
2 tbsp. unsalted butter, melted

8 oz. cream cheese, softened
¼ tsp. black pepper
½ tsp. garlic powder
2 (12 oz.) bags frozen corn, thawed

Preheat oven to 350 degrees. In a medium sized mixing bowl, combine mayonnaise, cream cheese, salt, pepper, onion powder, garlic powder, and ½ cup cheese. Beat at medium speed with electric mixer until smooth. Add corn and melted butter to mixing bowl; stir gently until combined. Spoon into 8x8 inch baking dish or 9-inch pie dish and top with remaining cheese. Bake for 20-25 minutes, or until cheese is bubbly. Serve warm with tortilla chips. This can also be made in a slow cooker! Prepare as directed, but spoon into slow cooker and set on low for 2-3 hours, high for 1-2 hours. Stir occasionally while cooking.

Pro-Tip: Make this a **Mexican Corn Dip** by using pepper jack cheese and substituting seasonings with 1 tablespoon taco seasoning.

Cucumber Bites *(6-8 servings)*

2 cucumbers
4 oz. cream cheese, softened
3 tbsp. ranch dressing
¼ tsp. Italian seasoning

12 cherry or grape tomatoes
1 tbsp. mayonnaise
¼ tsp. garlic salt
1 tbsp. fresh dill, minced

Peel cucumbers, rinse, and chop off ends. Slice into ½ inch rounds, scoop out a tiny bit of each center. In a small mixing bowl, combine cream cheese, mayonnaise, ranch, garlic salt, Italian seasoning, and fresh dill. Beat with electric mixer until well combined. Spoon filling into pastry bag with star tip and pipe 1 tablespoon filling on top of each cucumber slice. Slice tomatoes in half and press on top of each cucumber. Serve cold.

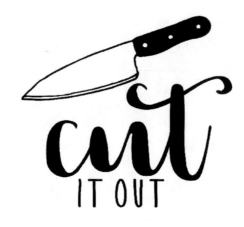

Deviled Eggs ǐ (24 pieces)

12 eggs

½ cup mayonnaise

1 tsp. Dijon mustard

1 tsp. salt, divided

¼ tsp. pepper

Put eggs and ½ teaspoon salt in a large pot with enough water to cover all the eggs. Heat the pot on high heat on the stove, bring to a rolling boil. Leave the pot on the burner but turn off the heat and place a cover on the pot. Let sit for 12-14 minutes. Take the pot off stove and run cold water into pot to cool eggs. Gently tap each egg on side of pot to create a crack, then peel shells off eggs. Cut each egg in half lengthwise, dump the egg yolks into a small mixing bowl. When all egg halves are emptied, smash up yolks with a fork and add mayonnaise, mustard, remaining salt, and pepper. Mix well. Spoon mixture into pastry bag and cut an opening on bag, pipe mixture into egg halves.

ǐ **Pro-Tip:** to make these extra pretty, use a cake decorating tip when piping into eggs and give a light sprinkle of paprika for some color.

Fruit Dip ǐ (8-10 servings)

4 oz. cream cheese, softened

1 cup frozen whipped topping, thawed

7 oz. marshmallow crème

In a medium sized mixing bowl, combine cream cheese and marshmallow crème. Beat with an electric mixer at medium speed for about 2 minutes, until smooth and creamy. Add whipped topping and continue to mix for another 2 minutes, store in refrigerator until serving. Serve with assorted fresh fruit or eat with a spoon if you really want to.

Fruity Mini Pancake Skewers ǐ (8-10 servings)

1 cup gluten-free baking mix (like Bisquick®)

½ cup milk

1 egg, beaten

1-pint fresh strawberries, sliced

2-3 bananas, sliced

1-pint fresh blueberries

confectioners sugar

maple syrup

In a medium size mixing bowl, whisk together baking mix, milk, and eggs. Heat an electric skillet or non-stick pan on medium heat. Spoon batter into squeeze bottle, squeeze a quarter-size amount of batter into pan. When the bubbles rise and bottom is golden, flip to other side to cook. When all pancakes are done, assemble skewers. Start with a pancake on the bottom, add 1 slice strawberry, 1 slice banana, another pancake, and repeat layering one more time. Add a fresh blueberry to top and place a skewer through the middle. Lightly dust with confectioners sugar and drizzle with maple syrup.

Guacamole ⅄ *(6-8 servings)*

4 avocados, halved and seeded
½ cup prepared pico de gallo
1 clove garlic, minced

2 tsp. lime juice
¼ - ½ tsp. salt (to taste)

Using a spoon, scoop avocado pulp out of skin and put in a medium sized mixing bowl. Add lime juice and mash pulp with a potato masher or fork until there are no large clumps. Add pico de gallo, garlic and salt; stir together well. Serve immediately, or store in refrigerator until ready to serve.

Storing Guacamole: To avoid turning brown, pack it tightly into a bowl with airtight lid, pressing out as many air bubbles as possible. Gently pour enough room temperature water on the top, covering with about ½ inch layer of water. Place lid on top. When ready to serve, gently pour water out and stir the guacamole.

How to find a ripe avocado: If the avocado is very firm, very green and the stem doesn't come off easily, it's not ready to eat. If the avocado is a dark green, slightly firm and the stem comes off easily and it's green underneath, it's ready to eat. If the avocado itself is very dark, smushy, and brown under the stem, it's yucky! Abort mission!

Homemade Queso ⅄ *(6-8 servings)*

12 oz. can evaporated milk
½ tsp. onion powder
½ tsp. salt

1 tbsp. cornstarch
¼ tsp. garlic powder
8 oz. grated pepper jack cheese

Combine evaporated milk, cornstarch, onion powder, garlic powder, and salt in a medium size sauce pan over low/medium heat and whisk together well. Bring to a light simmer (do not boil) and whisk frequently. Reduce heat to low and add half of cheese, stirring until completely melted. Add remaining cheese and stir again until melted, serve warm with tortilla chips.

⅄**Pro-Tip:** grating the cheese yourself will result in a smoother consistency queso.

Hot Crab Dip ⅄ *(8-10 servings)*

16 oz. chive and onion cream cheese, softened
1 lb. imitation crab meat

2 cups grated sharp cheddar
2 tbsp. heavy cream

Preheat oven to 350 degrees. In a medium size mixing bowl, combine the cream cheese, crab meat, cheese, and heavy cream. Using an electric mixer, beat at medium speed until well-combined, about 1-3 minutes. Spoon into an 8x8 inch baking dish and bake for 15-20 minutes, or until warm and bubbly. Spoon into bread bowl, sprinkle with a little extra cheese and serve warm.

Hot Sausage Dip 🍴 *(6-8 servings)*

1 lb. ground sausage
15.5 oz. jar salsa

8 oz. grated cheddar cheese

Cook sausage in a skillet on medium heat until fully cooked through and browned, drain. Turn on 1 ½ quart slow cooker to low setting. Combine all ingredients in slow cooker and stir. Cook for about 1 hour until mixture is warm. Stir halfway through and once again before serving. Turn setting to warm and serve with tortilla chips.

Hummus 🍴🍴 *(6-8 servings)*

15 oz. can chickpeas, rinsed and drained
¼ cup lemon juice
½ tsp. sea salt
2-3 tbsp. water

2 tbsp. extra-virgin olive oil
1 medium clove garlic, minced
½ cup tahini
½ tsp. ground cumin

Combine tahini and lemon juice in a food processor and process for one minute. Scrape the sides and bottom of the bowl, then process again for another 30 seconds. Add olive oil, garlic, cumin, and salt, process again for 30 seconds. Add half of the chickpeas, process for one minute. Scrape sides and bottom, add remaining chickpeas and water. Process for another 1-2 minutes, until thick and smooth. Serve with gluten-free crackers, pita bread, veggies, and/or tortilla chips.

Hush Puppies 🍴🍴 *(6-8 servings)*

1 cup gluten-free cornmeal
¾ cup gluten-free all-purpose flour
3 tbsp. granulated sugar
2 tsp. baking powder
1 tsp. salt
½ tsp. baking soda

½ tsp. chipotle powder
¼ tsp. garlic powder
¼ tsp. onion powder
½ cup milk
1 egg
vegetable oil, for frying

In a medium size mixing bowl, combine cornmeal, flour, sugar, baking powder, salt, baking soda, Cajun seasoning, garlic powder and onion powder, whisk together. Add milk and beaten egg, stir to combine. Using a cookie scoop, distribute about 1 tablespoon per hush puppy onto a parchment lined baking sheet and set in refrigerator. Heat at least 2 inches oil in a pan on medium heat. When oil is hot, fry hush puppies in batches for about 2-3 minutes, or until a light golden brown. Transfer to a plate lined with paper towels to catch excess grease, serve warm with softened butter.

🍴 **Pro-Tip:** for the true restaurant experience, serve with **Honey Butter**! Combine 1 cup softened butter with 3 tablespoons honey in a medium size mixing bowl, beat at medium speed until blended and creamy. Store in fridge for up to 2 weeks.

Italian Nachos ᵞ (12-14 servings)

1 large bag restaurant style nachos
1 lb. ground sausage
2 (15 oz.) jars gluten-free Alfredo Sauce
1 cup grated parmesan cheese

3 cups grated mozzarella cheese
1 cup diced tomatoes
1 cup sliced black olives
2 green onions, sliced

Preheat oven to 350 degrees. Pour half of nachos into 9x13 inch casserole dish, baking pan, or oven-safe platter. In a skillet, cook sausage until browned and fully cooked through. Drain and return to pan, add alfredo sauce and stir. Scoop half of sausage mixture on top of nachos. Sprinkle ½ cup parmesan and 1 ½ cups of mozzarella on top of sausage mixture, repeat layering. Bake in oven until cheese has melted, about 10 minutes. Serve immediately, top with tomatoes, olives, and green onions as a garnish.

Jalapeno Popper Dip ᵞ (8-10 servings)

8 oz. cream cheese, softened
1 cup sour cream
1 tsp. garlic powder
4 oz. diced jalapenos, drained

3 cups grated sharp cheddar cheese
1 cup gluten-free breadcrumbs
¼ cup butter, melted

Preheat oven to 350 degrees. In a medium size mixing bowl, combine cream cheese, sour cream, and garlic powder. Beat with electric mixer until well combined. Add diced jalapenos and cheddar cheese, beat again. Spread into an 8x8 inch square baking dish or 9-inch pie plate. In a bowl, toss together breadcrumbs and melted butter, spread on top of dip. Bake in oven for 15-20 minutes, until hot and golden. Serve warm with chips, gluten-free crackers, or Pita Points (p. 32).

Jalapeno Ranch Dip ᵞ (6-8 servings)

1 cup mayonnaise
½ cup sour cream
1 oz. packet Ranch dressing

½ cup cilantro, minced
1 cup pickled jalapenos, drained
½ cup buttermilk

Combine mayonnaise, sour cream, and Ranch dressing packet in a medium size mixing bowl and whisk together well. In a food processor, puree cilantro and pickled jalapenos. Add puree and buttermilk to ranch mixture, whisk again until smooth. Add more buttermilk for a thinner consistency. Store in refrigerator up to 5 days.

Key Lime Pie Dip (6-8 servings)

16 oz. cream cheese, softened
¼ cup half and half
Juice and zest of 2 limes

½ cup confectioners sugar
½ tsp. vanilla
green food coloring (optional)

In a medium size mixing bowl, combine all ingredients and beat with electric mixer until smooth and well-blended. Serve with gluten-free graham crackers, cookies, and/or pretzels.

Layered Cheesy Nachos (12-14 servings)

1 large bag restaurant style nachos
2 (12 oz.) cans gluten-free hot dog chili
2 (15.5 oz.) jars gluten-free queso dip

2 cups grated mozzarella cheese
2 cups grated sharp cheddar cheese
shredded lettuce and diced tomatoes

Preheat oven to 350 degrees. Pour half of nachos into 9x13 inch casserole dish, baking pan, or oven-safe platter. In a large saucepan, combine chili and queso dip. Cook on medium heat until mixture is combined and hot, stirring constantly. Scoop half of dip mixture on top of nachos. Sprinkle 1 cup of mozzarella and 1 cup cheddar on top of chili mixture, repeat layering. Bake in oven until cheese has melted, about 10 minutes. Top with optional lettuce and tomatoes as a garnish.

Mango Salsa (6-8 servings)

1 avocado, halved, peeled and diced
1 mango, peeled and diced
½ red onion, finely chopped

½ bunch cilantro, finely chopped
juice of 1 lime

Combine all ingredients in a small mixing bowl, toss together to combine. Serve immediately or cover and store in refrigerator for up to 3 days.

Mini Stuffed Peppers (6-8 servings)

8 oz. cream cheese, softened
1/3 cup mayonnaise
1 package mini sweet bell peppers (cut in half and deseeded)

1 cup grated sharp cheddar cheese
¼ cup real bacon bits

In a medium size mixing bowl, combine cream cheese and mayonnaise, beat with electric mixture until smooth. Add cheddar cheese and bacon bits, beat again until well-combined. Spoon mixture into bell pepper halves, chill in refrigerator for about 30 minutes before serving.

Mini Sausage Pancake Skewers ⚱ *(8-10 servings)*

1 cup gluten-free baking mix
½ cup milk
1 egg, beaten

1 lb. ground sausage
maple syrup

In a medium size mixing bowl, whisk together baking mix, milk, and eggs. Heat an electric skillet or non-stick pan on medium heat. Spoon batter into squeeze bottle, squeeze about a quarter-size amount of batter into pan. When the bubbles rise and bottom is golden, flip to other side to cook and set pancakes aside. Form sausages into 1-inch patties, or the same size as the mini pancakes. Cook in skillet until patties are cooked through, about 3 minutes on each side. Transfer to a plate lined with paper towels. When all sausages are done, assemble skewers. Start with a pancake on the bottom, add sausage, another pancake, and repeat layering one more time. Drizzle with maple syrup and serve warm.

Mini Pizzas ⚱ *(12 pizzas)*

6 gluten-free English muffins
14 oz. jar pizza sauce

1 ½ cups grated mozzarella cheese
4 oz. package mini pepperoni

Preheat oven to 350 degrees. Split each English muffin in half and lay each piece on a cookie sheet, split side up. Spread 1 tablespoon pizza sauce on each piece, followed by 2 tablespoons mozzarella cheese and 8-10 mini pepperoni slices. Bake for 12-15 minutes, or until cheese is melted. Serve warm.

Pro-Tip: for a variety of options, use different toppings for each pizza like plain cheese, sausage, bacon, peppers, onions, mushrooms, olives, etc.

Onion Dip ⚱ *(6-8 servings)*

1 ½ tbsp. dried minced onion
1 tsp. onion powder
½ tsp. dried parsley
1 tsp. fine sea salt

½ tsp. granulated sugar
¼ tsp. black pepper
8 oz. sour cream

In a small mixing bowl, combine all ingredients and whisk together well. Store in refrigerator for at least 30 minutes before serving.

Onion Rings 🍴 *(6-8 servings)*

1 large sweet onion
½ cup sour cream
½ tbsp. salt
¼ tsp. black pepper

1 cup buttermilk
1 cup gluten-free all-purpose flour
1 tsp. garlic powder
canola oil, for frying

Heat a Dutch oven or pot over medium heat with about 2-3 inches of oil. Slice onion into ½ inch rings, separate and set aside. In a small mixing bowl, whisk buttermilk and sour cream. In another bowl, whisk together flour, salt, pepper, and garlic powder. Dip each ring into milk mixture, then dredge in flour mixture. You can use a fork or tongs to transfer them from the wet bowl to dry bowl. Repeat process one more time before setting onion rings on a plate. When the oil is hot enough for the onion rings to sizzle, place 3-4 onion rings in a single layer in oil and cook for about 3 minutes, turning over halfway through until crispy and golden brown. Let cool on paper towels before serving.

Peanut Butter Pie Dip 🌷 *(12-14 servings)*

8 oz. cream cheese, softened
1 tsp. vanilla extract
8 oz. frozen whipped topping, thawed

½ cup creamy peanut butter
½ cup confectioners sugar

Combine all ingredients in a medium size mixing bowl, beat at medium speed with electric mixer until well-combined. Store in refrigerator until ready to serve with gluten-free graham crackers, cookies, and/or pretzels.

Pecan Cheese Spread (French Quarter) 🌷 *(6-8 servings)*

8 oz. cream cheese, softened
1 clove garlic, minced
¼ cup light brown sugar
½ tsp. Dijon mustard

1 tsp. grated sweet onion
¼ cup butter
1 tsp. gluten-free Worcestershire
1 cup pecans, finely chopped

In a small mixing bowl, combine cream cheese, onion, and garlic. Beat at medium speed with electric mixer until well combined. Spoon onto serving platter and set aside. In a saucepan, combine butter, brown sugar, Worcestershire, and mustard. Cook on medium/low heat until sugar is dissolved. Remove pan from heat and stir in pecans. Cool slightly before spreading on top of cream cheese mixture. Serve warm with gluten-free crackers.

Pita Points (12-14 servings)

½ cup olive oil
½ tsp. Greek seasoning

12 gluten-free pita bread rounds
½ tsp. sea salt

Preheat oven to 400 degrees. Line two baking sheets with parchment paper, set aside. In a small bowl, mix olive oil and Greek seasoning. Cut each piece of pita bread into 8 slices using a sharp knife. Place triangles in large mixing bowl, pour olive oil mixture on top and toss until well-combined. Sprinkle with salt, toss again. Spread into baking sheets (you won't be able to fit all of them unless you have big pans), place in oven to bake for about 7-8 minutes, or until slightly crispy. Serve with your choice of dips.

Pizza Dip (14-16 servings)

14 oz. jar pizza sauce
4 oz. package mini pepperoni

2 cups grated mozzarella cheese

Combine all ingredients in 1 ½ quart slow cooker and stir. Cook on high setting for 2-3 hours or until cheese is melted, stirring occasionally. Turn to warm, serve with gluten-free Garlic Bread (p. 218) or other gluten-free bread of your choice.

Pizzadillas (4-6 servings)

4 gluten-free tortillas
4 oz. pepperoni
2 cups grated mozzarella cheese

½ cup parmesan cheese
2 tsp. Italian seasoning
pizza sauce (for serving)

Heat an electric skillet to 300 degrees or a non-stick pan on medium heat on the stove. Spray the pan with cooking spray, then place a tortilla on top. Sprinkle about ½ cup cheese on the tortilla, followed by ½ teaspoon seasoning. Lay about 4-6 pepperoni on one side of the tortilla (since you'll be folding it over), cook for about two minutes. Pull up the side with no pepperoni slightly to check the bottom, using a pair of tongs. When the bottom is light golden, fold it over on top of the other half. Continue to cook for about 1 minute, just until the cheese is melted. Transfer finished pizzadilla to a plate to cool slightly before slicing with a pizza cutter. Serve warm with pizza sauce.

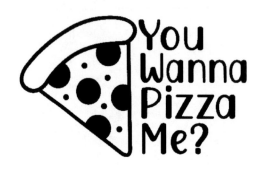

Pita Pizzas *(4 servings)*

4 slices gluten-free pita bread
1 cup pizza sauce

2 cups grated mozzarella cheese
pizza toppings (pepperoni, veggies, sausage)

Preheat oven to 375 degrees. Place pita bread slices on a large cookie sheet. Spread ¼ cup pizza sauce on each piece of bread. Sprinkle ½ cup grated mozzarella on top of pizza sauce. Sprinkle desired toppings onto each pizza; place pan in oven and bake for 10-12 minutes, until cheese is melted. Serve warm.

Potato Skins *(6-8 servings)*

6 small/medium russet potatoes
2 tbsp. olive oil
Sea salt
¼ cup unsalted butter

¼ tsp. onion powder
¼ tsp. garlic powder
1 cup grated sharp cheddar cheese
¼ cup real bacon bits

Preheat oven to 375 degrees. Rinse, dry, and poke holes around outside of potatoes using a fork. Rub the oil all around the potatoes, sprinkle generously with salt. Place potatoes on a baking sheet, bake for 50-60 minutes, until they are cooked through. Cool slightly so they're easy to handle. Increase oven temperature to 450 degrees. Cut potatoes in half lengthwise, use a spoon to scoop out the flesh. Leave ¼ - ½ inch around the inside of the skin. Melt butter in microwave, whisk in onion and garlic powders. Brush over tops and bottoms of the potatoes, place pans back in oven for 10 minutes. Flip potato skins over, top with cheese and bacon, bake for 10 minutes. Serve with Ranch or sour cream.

Pro-Tip: hang on to the cooked potato flesh to make some mashed potatoes!

Pretzel Turtles *(32 turtles)*

32 gluten-free mini pretzels
32 Rolos® (4 individual packages)

32 toasted or raw pecan halves

Preheat oven to 300 degrees. Line a cookie sheet with parchment paper, then lay pretzels on top of parchment paper. Place one Rolo® on top of each pretzel. Put cookie sheet in oven and bake for 4 minutes (the chocolate only needs to be soft enough to press a pecan into each one). Remove from oven, then immediately press one pecan into each piece of chocolate. This secures all three pieces together. Once they have cooled, store in airtight container at room temperature.

Pro-Tip: after doing some quick research about Rolos® containing gluten, they are considered to be gluten-free by the Hershey's company...with the exception of Rolo Minis. Remember to always check packaging and ingredients!

Pumpkin Pie Dip *(6-8 servings)*

2 cups confectioners sugar
8 oz. cream cheese, softened

15 oz. can pumpkin puree
1 tsp. pumpkin pie spice

Combine sugar and cream cheese in a medium size mixing bowl and beat at medium speed with electric mixer until smooth. Add pumpkin puree and pumpkin spice, continue mixing until smooth. Serve with gluten-free pretzels, gingerbread cookies, graham crackers, and/or apple slices.

Quesadilla Dip *(14-16 servings)*

1 lb. cooked fajita style chicken, diced
1 lb. Mexican blend grated cheese
16 oz. sour cream
¼ cup jalapeno juice*
2 tablespoons granulated sugar

½ tsp. cayenne pepper
½ tbsp. garlic powder
2 tbsp. paprika
2 tbsp. cumin

Preheat oven to 350 degrees. In a medium size mixing bowl, combine sour cream, jalapeno juice, sugar, cumin, paprika, garlic powder, and cayenne, whisk. Add chicken and Mexican cheese, stir together and spoon into 8x8 inch baking dish or 9-inch pie plate. Sprinkle mozzarella cheese on top and bake for 20-25 minutes, or until cheese is bubbly. Serve warm with tortilla chips.

Pro-Tip: keep a jar of jalapenos in your fridge. You can use the jalapenos, the juice, or all of it in different recipes.

Quesadilla Sauce *(6-8 servings)*

1 cup mayonnaise
2 tsp. cumin
½ tsp. cayenne
2 tbsp. jalapeno juice (from a can of jalapenos)

2 tsp. granulated sugar
2 tsp. paprika
½ tsp. garlic powder

Combine all ingredients in a small mixing bowl and whisk together well. Store in airtight container in refrigerator for up to 2 weeks. Serve with quesadillas or tacos.

This Quesadilla Sauce is one of those items that if I make Quesadillas at home and don't have this on hand, my husband says, "Where is the Quesadilla Sauce? We can't have Quesadillas without the sauce, that's illegal!" Although I tease him for being overdramatic, honestly I agree. It should be illegal. I also love adding this to tacos.

Ranch Dip *(6-8 servings)*

1 cup mayonnaise
1 tsp. dry chives
1 tsp. dry dill
1 tsp. onion powder
½ tsp. black pepper

½ cup sour cream
1 tsp. dry parsley
1 tsp. garlic powder
1 tsp. salt
2 tsp. gluten-free Worcestershire

Combine all ingredients in a small mixing bowl and whisk together well. Store in airtight container in refrigerator for up to 2 weeks.

Roasted Mixed Nuts *(14-16 servings)*

1 cup raw cashews
1 cup raw almonds
1 cup raw pecans

¼ cup olive oil
½-1 tsp. sea salt (to taste)

Preheat oven to 350 degrees. In a medium size mixing bowl, combine all nuts and olive oil, toss together well until nuts are evenly coated with oil. Spread into a lightly greased 9x13 inch baking dish, place in oven and bake for about 20 minutes, or until nuts are lightly roasted and fragrant. Remove from oven, sprinkle with salt and stir together with a spatula so they're evenly coated. Line a medium size mixing bowl with paper towels, dump nuts into bowl to let cool completely for at least 2 hours before serving. When nuts have cooled, store in an airtight container at room temperature.

Pro-Tip: for a different flavor, use melted butter and seasoned salt. You can also use different blends of nuts to mix it up, just make sure they're raw and haven't already been previously roasted.

Shrimp Dip *(8-10 servings)*

8 oz. cream cheese, softened
1 cup grated pepper jack cheese
1 tsp. gluten-free Worcestershire sauce
4 oz. can tiny shrimp, drained and chopped
Sliced green onions (garnish)

2 tsp. onion powder
1/3 cup mayonnaise
¼ cup sour cream
1 tsp. lemon juice

Preheat oven to 350 degrees. In a medium size mixing bowl, combine all ingredients (except green onions) and beat with electric mixer until well-combined. Spoon into a 1-quart baking dish, bake for about 20 minutes or until the cheese is melted and bubbly. Top with green onions, if desired. Serve warm with gluten-free crackers, chips, or Pita Points (p. 32).

Slow Cooker BBQ Meatballs 🍴 *(40 meatballs)*

30 oz. frozen gluten-free meatballs
18 oz. bottle honey BBQ sauce

1 cup ranch dressing
½ cup light brown sugar

Coat a 4-quart slow cooker with cooking spray, lay meatballs inside. In a small mixing bowl, whisk together BBQ sauce, ranch dressing, and light brown sugar. Pour on top of meatballs, cook on low for 2 hours until hot. Turn setting to warm and serve.

Spicy Bean Dip 🍴 *(6-8 servings)*

1 (20 oz) can refried pinto beans
5 slices canned jalapenos
½ tsp. onion powder
2-3 tbsp. brine from canned jalapenos

½ tsp. salt
½ tsp. sugar
1/8 tsp. cayenne pepper

Combine all ingredients in food processor, puree until smooth. Dip will be thick, add more brine for a thinner consistency. Cover and refrigerate for at least one hour before serving. Store in airtight container in refrigerator.

Spinach Artichoke Dip 🍴 *(8-10 servings)*

8 oz. cream cheese, softened
¼ cup sour cream
¼ cup mayonnaise
½ tsp. garlic powder

2/3 cup grated parmesan cheese
2/3 cup grated Monterey jack cheese
14 oz. can quartered artichoke hearts
6 oz. frozen spinach, thawed

Preheat oven to 350 degrees. Grease a 1-quart baking dish with cooking spray. In a medium size mixing bowl, combine cream cheese, sour cream, mayonnaise, garlic powder. Beat with electric mixer until smooth. Add parmesan and Monterey jack cheese, beat again until well-combined. Drain and chop both artichoke hearts and spinach, squeeze to drain excess liquid. Add chopped artichokes and spinach, stir together well and spread evenly into 8x8 inch baking dish. Bake for about 20 minutes, until hot and cheeses are melted. Serve with Pita Points (p. 32), tortilla chips, or gluten-free crackers.

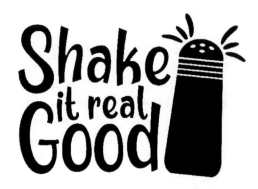

Spinach Dip ⍟ *(14-16 servings)*

1 oz. packet ranch dressing mix
10 oz. package frozen spinach, thawed

1 cup mayonnaise
16 oz. sour cream

In a medium mixing bowl, combine ranch dressing, mayonnaise and sour cream. Make sure you drain and squeeze as much water out of the spinach as possible to avoid the dip becoming soupy from the added liquid before adding to bowl. For a finer textured dip, chop spinach well. Add spinach into sour cream mixture and beat with electric mixture until well-combined. Chill for about 30 minutes before serving. Serve with cubes of beer bread and/or vegetables.

Stuffed Mushrooms ⍟⍟ *(12 mushrooms)*

12 whole fresh mushrooms
1 ½ tbsp. unsalted butter
1 tbsp. minced garlic

4 oz. cream cheese, softened
¼ cup grated parmesan cheese
¼ tsp. onion powder

Preheat oven to 350 degrees. Grease a baking sheet with cooking spray, set aside. Wipe off mushrooms with a clean damp paper towel, carefully remove stems and place mushroom caps on baking sheet. Chop stems into a fine consistency, discard the tough ends. Heat butter in a skillet on medium heat, add stems and cook until slightly tender. Add garlic, continue cooking until moisture has evaporated. In a medium size mixing bowl, combine cream cheese, parmesan, onion powder, and mushroom sauté. Beat with electric mixer until well-blended. Pipe into pastry bag and cut off tip, squeeze a heaping amount into each mushroom. Sprinkle with breadcrumbs, if desired. Place pan in oven to bake for about 20 minutes, serve warm.

⍟ **Pro-Tip:** this recipe can easily be converted to dairy-free by using dairy-free cream cheese and dairy-free parmesan *or* 1 tbsp. nutritional yeast.

Sweet Chex Mix ⍟ *(14-16 servings)*

12 oz. box Rice or Corn Chex® cereal
12 oz. bag semisweet chocolate chips
¾ cup creamy peanut butter

½ cup unsalted butter
1 tbsp. vanilla extract
6 cups confectioners sugar

Dump cereal into a large mixing bowl, set aside. In a large microwave safe bowl, combine chocolate chips, peanut butter, and butter. Microwave in 30 second intervals, stirring in between each interval until melted and smooth. Add vanilla and stir. Pour melted chocolate over cereal, gently stir together with a spatula and do not overmix. Add confectioners sugar, gently stir again until cereal is completely coated with sugar and do not overmix. Serve immediately or store in airtight container.

Sweet 'n Sour Meatballs 🍴 *(40 meatballs)*

30 oz. bag frozen gluten-free meatballs
12 oz. pineapple juice
6 oz. gluten-free soy sauce

6 oz. gluten-free teriyaki sauce
¾ cup light brown sugar

Place meatballs in slow cooker (at least 2 ½ quart size). Combine pineapple juice, soy sauce, teriyaki sauce, and sugar in a small mixing bowl. Whisk together and pour over top of meatballs in slow cooker. Turn on low setting and cook for 3-4 hours, stirring occasionally. Turn setting to warm to keep hot while serving.

Taco Dip 🍴 *(16-20 servings)*

8 oz. cream cheese, softened
8 oz. sour cream
20 oz. can refried pinto beans
1 oz. packet taco seasoning
15 oz. can black beans, rinsed and drained

16 oz. jar salsa
2 cups grated cheddar cheese
1 bag shredded lettuce
1 cup diced tomatoes

In a medium mixing bowl, combine taco seasoning, cream cheese, sour cream, and refried beans. Using an electric mixer, beat at medium speed for about 2 minutes until mixture is well-combined. Spread into bottom of a 9x13 inch baking dish and smooth into an even layer. Spoon black beans on top of bean mixture in dish, followed by salsa on top into an even layer. Sprinkle grated cheese on top, followed by bag of shredded lettuce and chopped tomatoes. Place plastic wrap over dish and store in refrigerator before serving with tortilla chips.

Three Cheese Chili Dip 🍴 *(14-16 servings)*

16 oz. cream cheese, softened
15 oz. can gluten-free chili

1 cup grated Monterey jack cheese
1 cup grated sharp cheddar cheese

Preheat oven to 350 degrees. Spread cream cheese on bottom of a 9x13 inch baking dish. Spoon chili on top of cream cheese in an even layer; sprinkle grated cheese on top of chili. Bake in oven until top layer of cheese is melted (about 10-15 minutes). Serve warm with tortilla chips.

🍴 **Pro-Tip:** use your favorite chili in this recipe, whether it's beans or meat! For a vegetarian version, use gluten-free vegetarian bean chili.

Trail Mix (14-16 servings)

4 cups Corn Chex® cereal
4 cups Rice Chex® cereal
1 cup raw mixed nuts
1 cup gluten-free pretzels
4 tsp. gluten-free Worcestershire sauce

¼ cup butter, melted
1 tsp. seasoned salt
½ tsp. garlic powder
½ tsp. onion powder

Preheat oven to 250 degrees. In a large mixing bowl, combine cereals, nuts, and pretzels, toss together to mix. In a small mixing bowl, whisk together butter, Worcestershire, and seasonings. Pour over cereal mix in large bowl, toss together to combine. Spoon mix into a large roasting pan, bake for 1 hour, stirring every 15 minutes. Spread onto paper towels or parchment paper to cool, store in airtight container.

Veggie Tray (8-10 servings)

1 head Broccoli
1 bag baby carrots
Dips (ranch, hummus, guacamole, etc.)

2 cucumbers
1 pint cherry tomatoes
1 bunch celery

Cut broccoli into bite-size florets. Peel and slice cucumbers into ½ inch thick rounds, cut off edges of celery and into 3–4-inch sticks. Arrange on a serving platter and serve with dips.

Pro-Tip: having a variety of dips for a veggie tray gives people options and they are more likely to indulge in the healthy goodness when they see a mini-buffet set up.

Zucchini Sticks (6-8 servings)

3 medium zucchini
2 eggs + 2 tbsp. water
¼ tsp. salt

¼ tsp. black pepper
½ cup grated parmesan cheese
1 cup gluten-free breadcrumbs

Preheat oven to 425 degrees. Line a baking sheet with parchment paper, set aside. Cut off ends of zucchini, then cut in half width wise, length wise, and quarter again (so you end up with 8 sticks from each zucchini). Beat the eggs and water in a shallow plate, add salt and pepper. In another shallow plate, toss together the breadcrumbs and parmesan cheese. Dip each zucchini stick in the egg wash, then roll through the breadcrumb mixture. Make sure each stick is fully covered with breadcrumbs, then set zucchini sticks on baking sheet. Place baking sheet in oven and bake for about 20 minutes, or until golden brown and crispy. Serve with ranch dressing.

Breakfast & Brunch

Apple Cider Donut Muffins 🍴 *(12 small muffins)*

2 cups gluten-free all-purpose flour
1 tbsp. baking powder
1 tsp. + 1 tbsp. cinnamon
½ tsp. salt
¼ tsp. nutmeg

¾ cup granulated sugar, divided
¼ cup light brown sugar
1 egg, beaten
1 cup apple cider, divided
½ cup vegetable oil

Preheat oven to 400 degrees. In a medium size mixing bowl, whisk together flour, baking powder, 1 teaspoon cinnamon, salt, nutmeg, and ½ cup granulated sugar and ¼ cup light brown sugar. Create a well in the center. Add oil, apple cider, and beaten egg. Stir together just until combined, batter will be lumpy. Distribute evenly into lined muffin pan, place in oven to bake for 20-24 minutes, or until a light golden brown. Remove pan from oven, transfer muffins to cooling rack to cool. In a small bowl, whisk together 1 tablespoon cinnamon and ¼ cup granulated sugar. Dip the top of each muffin first into ¼ cup apple cider, then into the cinnamon sugar mixture. Store muffins in airtight container for up to 3 days or wrap individually and store in freezer.

Apple Cider Donuts 🍴 *(12 donuts)*

2 cups gluten-free all-purpose flour
1 ½ cups granulated sugar, divided
½ cup light brown sugar
2 tsp. baking powder
1 tsp. + 1 tbsp. cinnamon
½ tsp. ground nutmeg

½ teaspoon salt
1 large egg, beaten
1 cup milk
¾ cup apple cider, divided
2 tbsp. butter, melted
2 tsp. vanilla

Preheat oven to 350 degrees, grease two donut pans with cooking spray and set aside. In a large mixing bowl, sift flour, baking powder, cinnamon, nutmeg, and salt. Whisk in 1 cup granulated sugar and light brown sugar. In a small mixing bowl, whisk together egg, milk, ¼ cup apple cider, butter, and vanilla. Pour the wet mixture into the dry mixture and stir together just until combined. Spoon batter into a pastry bag, snip off the end and squeeze into each donut cavity, a little over ¾ full. Bake for 16-18 minutes, until toothpick comes out clean. Let cool for 5 minutes in pan, then gently remove onto a baking pan. In a small mixing bowl, combine ½ cup granulated sugar and 1 tablespoon cinnamon, stir together well. Dip donuts in ½ cup apple cider, then into cinnamon sugar mixture.

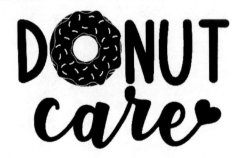

Apple Fritters (8-10 servings)

1 ½ cups gluten-free all-purpose flour
¼ cup granulated sugar
2 tsp. baking powder
½ tsp. salt
½ tbsp. cinnamon

1/3 cup milk
2 eggs, beaten
3 tbsp. applesauce
2 large Granny Smith apples
Canola or vegetable oil, for frying

In a medium size mixing bowl, whisk together flour, sugar, baking powder, and salt. Make a well in the center, then add milk, eggs, applesauce, and stir just to combine. Peel and finely chop or grate apples, add to batter and stir. Heat at least 2 inches oil in heavy skillet or Dutch oven on medium heat. Lightly drop about ¼ cup batter into oil, making sure to space out so they don't stick together. Cook on each side until golden brown, about 2 minutes. Using a slotted spoon, transfer fritters to paper towel lined plate to drain. For the glaze, whisk together 2 cups confectioners sugar and ¼ cup milk. Dunk each fritter into glaze on both sides, set on wire rack to drip and air dry.

Avocado Toast (2 servings)

2 slices gluten-free bread
1 ripe avocado

salt

Toast bread until golden and firm. Cut around the outside of the avocado, remove pit and scoop out flesh with a spoon. Spread onto both pieces of toast, lightly sprinkle with salt. Top with other chopped fresh vegetables, if desired.

Baked Breakfast Casserole (4-6 servings)

3 cups frozen shredded potatoes, thawed
½ cup real bacon bits
2 tbsp. butter, melted
1 cup grated sharp cheddar cheese

8 eggs, lightly beaten
1/3 cup milk
salt and pepper (to taste)

Preheat oven to 375 degrees. Spray 8x8 inch baking dish with cooking spray. Dump potatoes into baking dish and spread into even layer, then drizzle potatoes with melted butter. Sprinkle bacon bits over top of potatoes in baking dish, followed by grated cheese. In a medium mixing bowl, whisk together eggs and milk. Pour over bacon, cheese, and potatoes in baking dish, then sprinkle with desired salt and pepper. Bake for 45-50 minutes, until eggs are cooked through. Let set for 5 minutes, serve warm.

Pro-Tip: using thawed potatoes in this recipe makes a HUGE difference in the amount of baking time. Frozen potatoes will make you feel like you're watching paint dry while they bake since they take so much longer. Thawed potatoes rule!

Baked Oatmeal *(6-8 servings)*

1 ¾ cup milk
2 eggs, beaten
½ cup maple syrup
¼ cup applesauce
2 tsp. cinnamon
1 tsp. baking powder

2 tsp. vanilla
3 cups old fashioned oats
¼ tsp. salt
1 ½ cups frozen wild blueberries
1 cup slivered almonds

Preheat oven to 350 degrees. Combine milk, eggs, maple syrup, applesauce, cinnamon, baking powder, and vanilla in a large mixing bowl and whisk together well. Add oats and blueberries; stir together well. Spoon into a greased 11x7 inch casserole dish. Sprinkle almonds on top, bake for about 35 minutes. Serve warm, store leftovers in refrigerator for up to 7 days.

Pro-Tip: If preparing for on-the-go breakfast, spoon into glass containers and reheat in microwave for 30-60 seconds when ready to eat.

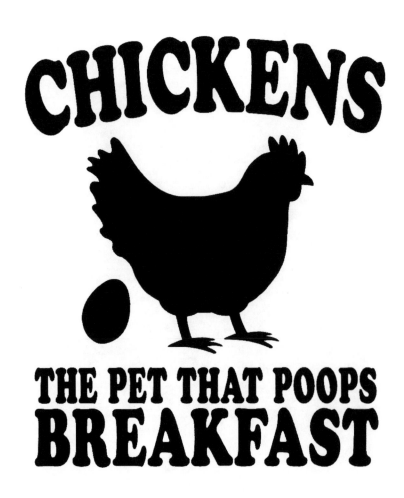

Banana Chocolate Chip Muffins ❦ *(16 small muffins)*

1 ½ cups gluten-free all-purpose flour
¾ cup granulated sugar
2 tsp. baking powder
1 tsp. baking soda
½ tsp. salt

3 very ripe bananas
1 egg
1 tsp. vanilla
¼ cup vegetable oil
½ cup mini chocolate chips

Preheat oven to 400 degrees. In a medium size mixing bowl or standing mixer, combine flour, sugar, baking powder, baking soda, and salt. In a blender, combine bananas, egg, vanilla, and oil. Puree until smooth. Pour banana puree into bowl with dry ingredients and beat at medium speed just until well combined, stir in chocolate chips. Fill up lined muffin pan about 2/3 full, place pan in oven to bake for about 20 minutes, until puffed up and golden brown. Remove pan from oven, transfer muffins to cooling rack to cool completely.

For the Chocolate Glaze ❦

1/3 cup confectioners sugar
1 tablespoon unsweetened dark cocoa

1-2 tbsp. water

Combine all ingredients in a small bowl and stir together until smooth, drizzle over cooled muffins.

Banana Oatmeal Bars ❦ *(16 bars)*

4 bananas, very ripe
1 cup oat milk
1 cup maple syrup

1 tsp. vanilla
5 cups old fashioned oats
¾ cup mini chocolate chips

Preheat oven to 350 degrees. Peel bananas, break into chunks and place in a blender with oat milk, maple syrup, and vanilla. Puree until smooth. Pour into a large mixing bowl, add oats and chocolate chips; stir together well. Spoon into a 9x13 inch pan that has been lined with parchment paper and press into an even layer. Bake for 35-40 minutes. Remove from oven and cool completely before cutting into bars. Wrap individually in plastic wrap, store in refrigerator for up to 5 days or in the freezer for up to 6 months. If freezing, pull out to thaw in refrigerator overnight.

❦ **Pro-Tip:** this is an item you can make variations depending on preferences. When I make a batch of these for my parents, I substitute chocolate chips with wild blueberries, add 1 tbsp. of cinnamon and add 1 cup of chopped walnuts. Feel free to experiment!

Banana Pancakes ⸙ *(4-6 servings)*

1 cup gluten-free all-purpose flour
1 tbsp. baking powder
¼ tsp. salt

¾ cup mashed ripe banana
1 large egg, beaten
¾ cup milk

In a medium size mixing bowl, combine flour, baking powder, and salt, whisk together and set aside. In a small mixing bowl, combine banana, egg, and milk, whisk vigorously. Pour wet ingredients into dry ingredients and whisk again, batter will be slightly lumpy. Heat a large skillet over medium heat, and coat with cooking spray. Pour ¼ cupfuls of batter onto the skillet and cook until bubbles appear on the surface. Flip with a flexible spatula and cook until lightly browned on the other side. Serve warm with maple syrup or spice it up with some Strawberry Maple Syrup (p. 69).

Blueberry Muffins ⸙ *(12 small muffins)*

2 cups gluten-free all-purpose flour
1 tbsp. baking powder
½ tsp. salt
¾ cup granulated sugar

½ cup vegetable oil
¾ cup milk
1 egg, beaten
1 cup frozen wild blueberries

Preheat oven to 400 degrees. In a medium size mixing bowl, whisk together flour, baking powder, salt, and granulated sugar. Create a well in the center. Add oil, milk, and beaten egg. Stir together just until combined, batter will be lumpy. Gently stir in blueberries. Distribute evenly into lined muffin pan, place in oven to bake for 20-24 minutes, or until a light golden brown. Remove pan from oven, transfer muffins to cooling rack to cool. Store muffins in airtight container for up to 3 days or wrap individually and store in freezer.

Bourbon Street Pancakes ⸙⸙ *(4-6 servings)*

½ cup butter
½ cup granulated sugar
½ cup light brown sugar
½ cup heavy cream

1 tbsp. dark rum
1 batch Buttermilk Pancakes (p. 49)
3-4 bananas, peeled and sliced
½ cup chopped pecans

In a medium saucepan, combine butter, both sugars, heavy cream, and dark rum. Bring to a simmer over medium heat for 2-4 minutes, stirring occasionally until it thickens and coats the back of a spoon. Remove from heat for about 30 minutes, it will thicken more as it cools. Make pancakes, layer with sliced bananas and chopped pecans, serve with rum sauce in place of maple syrup.

> *I saw this on a menu in a brunch restaurant, and about fell over when I read the description. My lower lip poked out when I realized this wasn't gluten-free, so the rebel in me decided to come home and make a version that I could eat.*

Breakfast Cups (12 servings)

12 large eggs
Salt and pepper, to taste
¾ cup fresh spinach, roughly chopped

¾ cup real bacon bits
¾ cup grated cheddar cheese

Preheat oven to 350 degrees. Spray 12-cavity muffin pan with nonstick cooking spray. In a medium size mixing bowl, beat eggs well. Add salt and pepper. Pour egg mixture into muffin cavities, filling halfway up. Top each cavity with spinach, bacon, and cheese. Bake for 15-20 minutes, or until set.

Breakfast Pizza (6-8 servings)

½ batch Pizza Dough (p. 223)
4.5 oz. real bacon bits
2 cups grated sharp cheddar

8 large eggs
1/3 cup half and half
¼ teaspoon black pepper

Preheat oven to 375 degrees. Coat a 12-inch round cake pan with cooking spray, press the pizza dough into the pan to form a crust. Sprinkle bacon on top of the crust, then grated cheese. In a medium mixing bowl, combine eggs, milk, and pepper. Whisk together well, pour over crust. Bake for 25-30 minutes, cut into slices and serve warm.

Breakfast Potatoes (4-6 servings)

3 large russet potatoes
¼ cup olive oil

½ teaspoon salt

Preheat oven to 375 degrees. Peel potatoes and cut into ½ inch cubes. Combine with olive oil in a medium size mixing bowl, toss together to coat evenly. Grease a baking pan with cooking spray, spread potatoes onto pan. Bake for 35-40 minutes, gently moving around with a spatula halfway through baking process. Remove pan from oven when potatoes are golden brown, sprinkle with salt and serve.

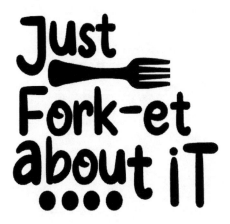

Just Fork-et about iT

Breakfast Quesadilla ❦ (1 serving)

1 gluten-free tortilla
1 large egg
Salt and pepper (to taste)

¼ cup grated cheddar cheese
2 tbsp. real bacon bits

Heat a non-stick skillet pan over low heat. Crack egg open into a bowl, beat with a fork. Pour egg into pan and spread to be about the same size as the tortilla, sprinkle with salt and pepper. When egg is nearly cooked through, sprinkle cheese on top, then cover with tortilla. Using a large spatula, slide under the egg and quickly flip over so the tortilla is now on the bottom. Sprinkle bacon bits on top, continue cooking until tortilla is lightly browned. Fold the tortilla over in half. When tortilla is done cooking, transfer to plate and cut into slices with pizza cutter. Serve immediately.

Breakfast Quiche ❦ (6-8 servings)

2 cups milk
6 eggs
1 cup gluten-free baking mix
½ cup grated parmesan cheese

¼ cup butter, softened
2 cups grated cheddar cheese
1 cup diced ham
½ tsp. salt

Preheat oven to 375 degrees. In a medium mixing bowl, combine milk, eggs, baking mix, butter, and parmesan. Using an electric mixer, beat at medium speed for about 1 minute. Stir in ham, cheddar, and salt. Grease a 9-inch round pie plate or 8x8 inch square baking dish with cooking spray. Pour ingredients into baking dish, place in oven to bake for 50-60 minutes, or until eggs are set. Remove dish from oven, let quiche sit for 10 minutes before serving. Store leftovers in refrigerator for 5 days.

Breakfast Sandwiches ❦ (4 servings)

4 gluten-free Cheddar Biscuits (p. 50), English muffins, or Buttermilk Biscuits (p. 49)
4 cooked sausage patties, oven baked bacon, or deli ham

Slice biscuits in half, place meat of choice in between pieces of biscuit. Feel free to add a slice of cheese, scrambled eggs, or you can make a meat-lover's version by piling on all three meats AND a slice of cheese with eggs. Pop in the microwave for 15-30 seconds when ready to eat or wrap them individually with plastic wrap and store in freezer. When ready to eat, pull a sandwich out of the freezer to thaw overnight in fridge, heat for 30 seconds when ready to serve.

Buttermilk Drop Biscuits *(12 biscuits)*

2 cups gluten-free all-purpose flour
2 tsp. baking powder
½ tsp. baking soda
1 tsp. granulated sugar

¾ tsp. salt
1 cup buttermilk
½ cup butter, melted

Preheat oven to 425 degrees, line a baking sheet with parchment paper and spray lightly with cooking spray. In a medium size mixing bowl, whisk together flour, baking powder, baking soda, sugar, and salt. In a small mixing bowl, combine buttermilk and melted butter, stir. Pour buttermilk mixture into flour mixture, gently stir together with a spatula just until combined. Drop ¼ cup of dough onto baking sheet, about 2 inches apart from each other. Bake until the biscuits are golden brown, about 13-15 minutes.

Buttermilk Pancakes *(20-22 pancakes)*

3 cups gluten-free all-purpose flour
¼ cup granulated sugar
1 tbsp. baking powder
2 tsp. baking soda
1 tsp. salt

2 eggs
3 cups buttermilk
¼ cup butter, melted
2 tsp. vanilla

Combine flour, sugar, baking powder, baking soda, and salt in a medium size mixing bowl, whisk together. In a small mixing bowl, whisk eggs, vanilla, butter, and buttermilk. Pour the wet ingredients into the flour mixture and whisk until most lumps are gone. Heat a large skillet over medium heat, coat with cooking spray. Pour ¼ cupfuls of batter onto the skillet and cook until bubbles appear on the surface. Flip with a flexible spatula and cook until lightly browned on the other side. Serve warm with butter, maple syrup, and a big smile.

I make these in big batches because our family eats them on a daily basis for breakfast. I do make these dairy-free and do so simply by replacing the buttermilk with oat milk (that curdles with vinegar) and plant butter. My daughter loves it when I throw in a few mini chocolate chips, and my son loves wild blueberries in his. We love the options.

Cappuccino Smoothie *(1 serving)*

12 oz. brewed coffee, cooled
1 scoop vanilla protein powder

1 cup plain yogurt
1 cup ice

Combine all ingredients in a blender and puree until smooth, serve immediately.

Cheddar Buttermilk Biscuits (12 biscuits)

2 cups gluten-free all-purpose flour
1 tbsp. granulated sugar
1 tbsp. baking powder
2 tsp. garlic powder
½ tsp. onion powder

½ tbsp. sea salt
1 cup buttermilk
½ cup unsalted butter, melted
1 ½ cups grated sharp cheddar cheese
¼ cup sour cream

Preheat oven to 400 degrees. In a medium size mixing bowl, whisk together flour, sugar, baking powder, garlic powder, onion powder, and salt. Add buttermilk, melted butter, sour cream, and cheddar cheese. Beat with electric mixer at medium speed just until combined, do not overmix. Using a 4 oz. cookie scoop (or 1/4 cup), distribute dough to a lined cookie sheet about 3 inches apart. Brush with more melted butter, if desired. Place pan in oven and bake for 20 minutes, or until light golden. Remove pan from oven and serve warm with butter.

Chicken and Waffles (4-6 servings)

1 bag frozen gluten-free chicken tenders
1 batch Waffles (p. 70)

maple syrup

Cook chicken tenders according to package directions (whether frying or baking). While chicken tenders are cooking, prepare one batch of waffles. Place 2 chicken tenders on top of each waffle, drizzle with maple syrup and serve warm.

Chocolate Donuts (8-10 donuts)

1 cup gluten-free all-purpose flour
¼ cup dark cocoa
1/3 cup granulated sugar
1 tsp. baking powder
½ tsp. salt
1 large egg, beaten

½ cup whole milk
2 tbsp. butter, melted
1 tsp. vanilla
¾ cup confectioners sugar
2 tbsp. dark cocoa
2-3 tbsp. milk

Preheat oven to 350 degrees, grease two donut pans with cooking spray and set aside. In a medium size mixing bowl, combine flour, ¼ cup cocoa, sugar, baking powder, and salt, whisk together. Add egg, milk, butter, and vanilla, whisk together until well combined. Spoon batter into a large pastry bag, cut about 1 inch off the tip of the bag. Pipe batter into donut pan about ¾ full, then place in oven and bake for 14-16 minutes (or until donut springs back lightly when touched). Remove from oven and turn donuts out of pan onto a parchment paper lined cookie sheet. Stir together confectioners sugar, 2 tablespoons cocoa and 2-3 tablespoons milk. Dip each donut in glaze, return to parchment paper to cool and set. Top with sprinkles, if desired.

Chocolate Peanut Butter Banana Smoothie *(1 serving)*

1 banana (cut into chunks and frozen)
1 scoop vanilla protein powder

1 tbsp. peanut butter
12 oz. chocolate almond milk

Combine all ingredients in a blender and puree until smooth, serve immediately.

Cinnamon Roll Muffins *(11 jumbo muffins)*

1 box King Arthur® gluten-free cake mix
1 small box Jell-O® instant vanilla pudding mix
¾ cup vegetable oil
½ cup whole milk
4 eggs
1 cup sour cream

1 tsp. ground cinnamon
¼ cup granulated sugar
1 tbsp. ground cinnamon
1 cup confectioners sugar
2-3 tbsp. milk

Preheat oven to 450 degrees. In a standing mixer or medium size mixing bowl, combine cake mix, pudding mix, 1 tsp. cinnamon, oil, milk, eggs, and sour cream. Beat with electric mixer at medium speed for 1-2 minutes, until well-combined. Line 2 jumbo muffin pans with liners, distribute half of batter evenly into cavities, about 1/3 full. In a small mixing bowl, combine granulated sugar and 1 tbsp. cinnamon, toss together until combined, then sprinkle evenly over each muffin. Spoon remaining batter on top of each muffin. Place pans in oven and bake for 11 minutes. Reduce oven temperature to 350 degrees, continue baking for another 17-18 minutes, or until toothpick inserted in muffins comes out clean. Remove pans from oven and let cool for about 5 minutes before removing muffins from pans and cooling completely on cooling racks. Combine confectioners sugar, vanilla, and milk in a small mixing bowl and stir together to combine. Spread evenly over top of each muffin and serve.

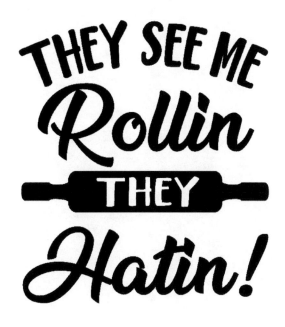

Cinnamon Rolls 🍴 *(12 servings)*

½ cup granulated sugar
1 cup milk (110-115 degrees)
1 tbsp. instant/rapid yeast
¼ cup unsalted butter, melted and cooled
2 large eggs, room temperature
1 tsp. apple cider vinegar
3 ¼ cups gluten-free all-purpose flour

2 tsp. baking powder
½ tsp. salt
½ cup half and half
¼ cup unsalted butter, softened
1 cup light brown sugar
2 tbsp. cinnamon

Preheat oven to 350 degrees. In a standing mixer, combine granulated sugar, warmed milk, and yeast. Cover with a kitchen towel and let it bubble up for about 2-3 minutes. Beat eggs in a small bowl before adding to large mixing bowl along with melted butter and apple cider vinegar. Add flour, baking powder, and salt to bowl. Using paddle attachment, mix for 1-2 minutes, until fully combined. Change paddle attachment to dough hook, mix on medium speed for 3-5 minutes. Transfer dough to a greased glass or metal bowl. Wet hands with warm water, rub the dough to make it smooth. Cover bowl with plastic wrap and set inside a larger bowl. Pour hot water inside larger bowl, surrounding the bowl with dough (this helps it rise). Cover both bowls with a kitchen towel and let rise for 20 minutes. In a small bowl, toss together light brown sugar and cinnamon, set aside. Lay a large piece of parchment paper on flat surface and grease with cooking spray. Place dough on top, sprinkle with extra gluten-free flour or rice flour, roll out dough using a rolling pin to ½ inch thick and into a 12x14 inch rectangle. Spread softened butter evenly on top, then sprinkle brown sugar cinnamon mixture over butter and press down. Use the edge of the parchment paper to fold the longest end up to start the roll. Roll the dough up tightly to form a log. Cut the log in half, then cut each half into six rolls using dental floss. Grease a 9x13 inch baking dish with cooking spray, then place the rolls inside. Heat half and half in microwave for 30 seconds before pouring on top of rolls. Bake rolls for 20-25 minutes, until light golden brown. Cool slightly before spreading icing on top and serve warm.

Cream Cheese Glaze 🥄

8 oz. cream cheese, softened
2 tbsp. butter, softened

2 cups confectioners sugar
1 tsp. vanilla

In a medium size mixing bowl, combine cream cheese and butter. Beat with electric mixer at medium speed for 2 minutes, then add confectioners sugar and vanilla. Continue beating for another 2 minutes. Set aside until ready to spread on rolls.

A bakery that was at a local farmer's market used to make these with blueberries as the filling, and they were incredible. To make that version of these rolls, substitute the butter/cinnamon/sugar filling with blueberry fruit spread or mashed fresh blueberries. Like strawberries instead of blueberries? Go for it! Chopped apples and cinnamon? Yes!! I love having a variety of options.

Cinnamon Toast 🍴 *(2 servings)*

4 pieces gluten-free bread
2 tbsp. softened butter

¼ cup granulated sugar
1 tbsp. ground cinnamon

Set oven to (high) broil. Spread ½ tablespoon of butter on each piece of bread, set each piece on a baking sheet. In a small bowl, stir together the cinnamon and sugar until well combined. Sprinkle 1 tsp. mixture on top of each piece of bread. Place baking sheet in oven and broil for 1-2 minutes, remove from oven and serve warm.

Crepes 🍴 *(12 servings)*

1 ¾ cups gluten-free flour*
¼ tsp. salt
3 eggs, room temperature

2 tbsp. butter, melted
2 cups milk, room temperature

In a large mixing bowl, whisk together flour and salt, create a well in the center. In another bowl, whisk eggs, butter, and milk. Pour wet ingredients into dry ingredients, whisk together very well. Transfer batter to a large measuring cup with a spout. Heat a 9-inch non-stick skillet pan on medium heat. Grease lightly with cooking spray. Hold skillet just above the heat, pour ¼ cup batter into pan and swirl to distribute evenly across flat surface of the pan. Cook until edges are lightly golden brown, about 90 seconds. Using a wide spatula, turn over and cook on other side until lightly golden brown, about 30 seconds. Transfer to a parchment-paper lined plate. Repeat process with remaining batter. Serve plain or spread Cream Cheese Icing (p. 215) in each crepe and roll up, then serve with Strawberry Maple Syrup (p. 69.).

🍴 **Pro-Tip:** for this recipe, be sure to use flour that does not contain xanthan gum. For best results, cover the bowl after making batter and let sit in refrigerator overnight.

Coastal Omelet 🍴 *(1 serving)*

3 eggs
¼ tsp. salt
1 tbsp. unsalted butter

¼ cup grated Monterey jack cheese
¼ cup cooked crab meat (no shells)
2 green onions, sliced

Combine eggs and salt in a bowl and beat well with a fork. Heat a small nonstick skillet pan over medium heat, melt butter. Once the butter is melted, add eggs to skillet and immediately reduce heat to low. Using a spatula, gently pull the cooked eggs to the center, letting the liquid egg fill in the space behind it. Continue this process until the eggs are almost set. When the omelet slides around the pan easily and you can slide a spatula underneath it, flip the omelet over and remove from heat. Sprinkle cheese on top along with crab and green onions, then fold omelet over in half and transfer to plate to serve warm.

Coffee Cake ▼ (12-16 servings)

1 box King Arthur® gluten-free cake mix
1 small box Jell-O® instant vanilla pudding mix
¾ cup vegetable oil
½ cup whole milk
4 eggs
1 cup sour cream

¼ cup granulated sugar
1 tbsp. cinnamon
1 cup gluten-free all-purpose flour
1 cup light brown sugar
1 tsp. cinnamon
½ cup butter, melted

Preheat oven to 350 degrees. In a medium size mixing bowl, combine cake mix, pudding mix, oil, milk, egg, and sour cream. Beat with electric mixer at medium speed for 1 minute, until well combined. Spoon half of batter into a greased 9x13 inch baking dish. In a small bowl, toss together granulated sugar and 1 tablespoon cinnamon, sprinkle evenly on top of batter. Cover with remaining batter. In a small mixing bowl, combine flour, light brown sugar, 1 teaspoon cinnamon, and melted butter. Toss together until combined, then sprinkle on top of batter. Bake for 35-40 minutes, until toothpick in center comes out clean. Cool slightly before cutting into slices and serve.

Crab Cake Benedict ▼▼ (4 servings)

4 Crab Cakes (p. 168)
2 gluten-free English muffins
1 tsp. vinegar

4 eggs
Hollandaise Sauce (p. 87)

Split muffins into two, toast and set aside, place one crab cake on top of each one. Fill a medium size pot with water about 3 inches deep. Bring water to a boil, then reduce to a simmer. Add 1 teaspoon vinegar to water, this helps egg white stay together while cooking. Break eggs one at a time into a small cup, lower egg gently into the water. Cook eggs in water for 3-5 minutes, depending on how soft you like the yolk. Remove egg with a slotted spoon and place on top of crab cake. Top with Hollandaise Sauce and serve warm.

Creamy Grits ▼ (6-8 servings)

1 cup stone ground grits
2 cups water
2 cups half and half

¼ cup butter
½ tsp. salt

Combine grits, chicken broth, and half and half in a pot on medium/high heat and stir together. Bring to a boil, then reduce heat to low/medium, cover and cook for about 20 minutes, stirring occasionally. When grits have thickened and are cooked through, add butter and salt, stir together and cover again until butter has melted. Stir and serve.

Crunchy Granola (Cereal) ♟ *(6-8 servings)*

4 cups old-fashioned gluten-free oats
½ cup chopped walnuts
1 cup pumpkin seeds
¾ tsp. salt

½ tsp. cinnamon
½ cup melted coconut oil
½ cup maple syrup
1 tsp. vanilla

Preheat oven to 350 degrees, line a large baking sheet with parchment paper and set aside. Combine the oats, nuts, seeds, salt, and cinnamon in a large mixing bowl and stir together to blend. Pour in the oil, syrup, and vanilla, stir together well so that oats, nuts, and seeds are evenly coated. Spread granola onto a large, greased baking sheet in an even layer. Place pan in oven and bake until lightly golden, about 27-28 minutes. Remove pan from oven, let granola cool completely. Break into pieces if desired, transfer to an airtight container and store at room temperature for up to 2 weeks or in sealed freezer bags for up to 3 months in the freezer.

If a fly on the wall heard me refer to "the greatest cereal in the world" in my house, I would be referring to this cereal. I love to eat this in a bowl with oat milk and a huge smile on my face. It's the breakfast of champions. Maybe one day I'll be a champion.

Danish Pastries 🍴🍴🍴 *(6-8 servings)*

2 cups gluten-free all-purpose flour
½ cup granulated sugar
1 packet instant yeast
½ cup butter, cubed and softened
¾ cup milk
½ tsp. vanilla

1 tsp. salt
2 eggs, separated
½ cup jam or cream cheese
½ cup confectioners sugar
2 tsp. water

Preheat oven to 400 degrees. In a freezer-safe mixing bowl, stir together flour, sugar, and yeast. Add the butter and cut into flour mixture using a pastry cutter, fork, or pulse in a food processor until it looks like small peas. In another mixing bowl, whisk together milk, vanilla, egg yolks, and salt until well combined. Pour liquid mixture into flour mixture, stir until fully combined and dough is very sticky. Cover with plastic wrap and place in freezer for 30 minutes. Sprinkle 1 tablespoon flour onto a large piece of parchment paper, remove dough from freezer and place on top. Dust the dough with 1 more tablespoon flour, gently fold over itself three times. Using your hands, form a dough round that is about 7 inches in diameter and 1 inch thick. Using a greased 3-inch biscuit cutter, press straight down to cut circles of dough. Transfer dough rounds to a parchment-lined baking sheet, cover with plastic wrap and a kitchen towel, then let rise for 30 minutes. Grease the back of a rounded tablespoon with cooking spray, press down in center of each piece of dough. Fill center with jam or softened cream cheese. Whisk 1 tablespoon water with egg whites, then brush over top of each piece of dough. Place pan in oven to bake for 18-20 minutes, or until a light golden brown. Remove pan from oven, let danishes cool for about 15 minutes. Stir together confectioners sugar and water, drizzle on top of each one and serve. Store leftovers in an airtight container.

Double Chocolate Muffins *(12 muffins)*

1 ½ cups gluten-free all-purpose flour
½ cup unsweetened cocoa
1 tbsp. baking powder
½ tsp. salt
¾ cup granulated sugar

½ cup vegetable oil
¾ cup milk
1 egg, beaten
1 cup chocolate chips

Preheat oven to 400 degrees. In a medium size mixing bowl, whisk together flour, cocoa, baking powder, salt, and granulated sugar. Create a well in the center. Add oil, milk, and beaten egg. Stir together just until combined, batter will be lumpy. Gently stir in chocolate chips. Distribute evenly into lined muffin pan, place in oven to bake for 20-24 minutes. Remove pan from oven, transfer muffins to cooling rack to cool. Store muffins in airtight container for up to 3 days.

Eggs Benedict *(4 servings)*

2 gluten-free English muffins
4 slices Canadian Bacon
4 eggs

1 tsp. vinegar
Hollandaise Sauce (p. 87)

Split muffins into two, toast and set aside, place one piece of Canadian Bacon on top of each one. Fill a medium size pot with water about 3 inches deep. Bring water to a boil, then reduce to a simmer. Add 1 tsp. vinegar to water, this helps egg white stay together while cooking. Break eggs one at a time into a small cup, lower egg gently into the water. Cook eggs in water for 3-5 minutes, depending on how soft you like the yolk. Remove egg with a slotted spoon and place on top of Canadian Bacon. Top with Hollandaise Sauce and serve warm.

French Toast Casserole *(6-8 servings)*

1 lb. loaf gluten-free bread
6 large eggs
2 cups milk
1 tsp. vanilla extract

1 cup butter, melted
1 cup light brown sugar
2 tbsp. maple syrup
2 tsp. ground cinnamon

Coat a 9x13 inch baking dish with cooking spray. Arrange slices of bread in two rows, overlapping the slices. In a medium size mixing bowl, combine the eggs, milk, and vanilla. Beat with whisk until well blended. Pour liquid over the bread slices in baking dish, making sure all pieces of bread are covered evenly. Spoon some of the liquid in between the slices. Cover with foil and refrigerate overnight. In the morning, remove baking dish from refrigerator and preheat oven to 350 degrees. Combine butter, brown sugar, maple syrup, and cinnamon in a small mixing bowl and whisk together until well combined. Pour topping over the casserole, place dish in oven, and bake for 40 minutes, or until puffed and lightly golden. Serve warm.

French Toast Waffles *(4 servings)*

8 slices gluten-free bread
4 eggs
½ cup milk

1 tsp. cinnamon
1 tbsp. granulated sugar
2 tbsp. butter, melted

In a small mixing bowl, whisk together eggs, milk, cinnamon, and sugar. Slowly pour in melted butter, whisk again to combine. Turn on waffle maker, spray plates with cooking spray. When waffle maker indicates it's ready, take one piece of bread and dip it in the egg mixture, both sides. Immediately place it in the waffle maker, close the lid, then check on it after about a minute. When it's lightly browned and golden, you know it's ready. Remove from waffle maker, repeat process with remaining pieces of bread. Smother each one as desired with maple syrup.

Fruit Smoothie *(1 serving)*

12 oz. water or almond milk   1 scoop vanilla protein powder
1 cup frozen fruit (blueberries, strawberries, etc.)

Combine all ingredients in a blender and puree until smooth. Serve immediately.

This is my favorite way to slip some fiber and protein into my kids' bellies without them suspecting anything. Grocery stores typically carry a variety of frozen fruits to choose from, and one of my personal favorite fruits to use in smoothies is frozen bananas. Just slice some almost-ripe bananas and put them in individual freezer bags to grab as a quick and easy option. Using frozen fruit in these smoothie recipes gives them the consistency of a slushie or milkshake! My favorite protein powders to use in smoothies are plant-based as well to cut down on dairy consumption since too much of it destroys my sinus congestion, ocular migraines and my sensitive tummy issues.

Garden Frittata *(4 servings)*

1 tbsp. olive oil
¾ cup broccoli florets
1 red bell pepper, seeded and diced
¼ cup diced onion

4 eggs
½ cup egg whites
½ cup grated cheddar cheese
salt and pepper to taste

Preheat oven to 400 degrees. Heat oil in an oven-safe 8-inch pan on medium heat. Add onion and pepper to pan, cook until tender, about 3-4 minutes. Add broccoli to pan with 1 tablespoon water and continue cooking until broccoli is tender. Season vegetables with salt and pepper, transfer to a bowl. Wipe pan with a paper towel, then coat with cooking spray. In a medium mixing bowl, combine eggs and egg whites, whisk together well. Add vegetables and cheese, stir to combine before spooning back into pan. Bake in oven for 15-18 minutes, until eggs are set. Cool slightly before cutting into wedges and serve.

Glazed Donuts ♔ *(12 donuts)*

2 cups gluten-free all-purpose flour
¾ cup granulated sugar
2 tsp. baking powder
1 tsp. salt
¾ cup milk

2 large eggs, room temperature
2 tsp. vanilla
½ cup vegetable oil
¾ cup confectioners sugar
2-3 tbsp. milk

Preheat oven to 425 degrees, grease two donut pans with cooking spray and set aside. In a large mixing bowl, combine flour, sugar, baking powder, and salt, whisk together well. In a small mixing bowl, combine ¾ cup milk, eggs, vanilla, and oil, whisk together. Pour wet ingredients into bowl with dry ingredients, whisk just until combined. Spoon batter into a large pastry bag, cut about 1 inch off the tip of the bag. Pipe batter into donut pan about ¾ full, then place in oven and bake for 8-10 minutes, until the donuts rise and are light golden brown. Carefully remove donuts from pan and transfer to a cooling rack with parchment paper underneath. In a small mixing bowl, stir together confectioners sugar and milk until smooth. When donuts have cooled, dip top into glaze and set on cooling rack. Repeat 1-2 more times until glaze is white. Store donuts in airtight container for 3 days.

Greek Scrambled Eggs ♔ *(1 serving)*

1 tbsp. olive oil
1 clove garlic, minced
½ cup diced tomatoes

3 eggs, beaten
salt and pepper to taste
¼ cup feta cheese

Heat oil on medium heat in a non-stick skillet pan. Add garlic and tomatoes, cook just until fragrant. Pour eggs into pan and reduce heat to low/medium, stirring occasionally and cook until eggs are cooked through. Sprinkle with salt and pepper, spoon eggs onto a plate. Sprinkle feta cheese on top, serve immediately.

Green Eggs and Ham Omelet ♔ *(1 serving)*

3 eggs
¼ tsp. salt
1 tbsp. unsalted butter

¼ cup grated sharp cheddar
¼ cup diced ham
¼ cup pesto

Combine eggs and salt in a bowl and beat well with a fork. Heat a small nonstick skillet pan over medium heat, melt butter. Once the butter is melted, add eggs to skillet and immediately reduce heat to low. Using a spatula, gently pull the cooked eggs to the center, letting the liquid egg fill in the space behind it. Continue this process until the eggs are almost set. When the omelet slides around the pan easily and you can slide a spatula underneath it, flip the omelet over and remove from heat. Sprinkle cheese on top along with ham, then fold omelet over in half and transfer to plate. Spread with pesto and serve immediately.

Green Protein Smoothie ⍾ *(1 serving)*

12 oz. water
1 cup organic frozen blueberries
1 scoop vanilla protein powder

2 tbsp. hemp protein
2 large handfuls juicing greens

Combine all ingredients in a blender and puree for at least 1 minute, until smooth. Serve in a large 24 oz. cup and drink immediately.

⍾**Pro-Tip:** here is another option for variety. Change up your frozen fruit, protein, and even types of greens to make sure your body is getting the nutrients it needs. Smoothies are typically easy on the digestive system since it doesn't have to work so hard on digesting since everything is already pureed.

Hashbrown Patties ⍾ *(servings)*

3 cups frozen shredded potatoes, thawed
¼ cup gluten-free all-purpose flour
½ tsp. salt

1 egg, beaten
vegetable oil, for frying

Combine hashbrown potatoes, flour, salt, and egg in a medium size mixing bowl and stir together well. Using hands, form into ½ cup size patties and place on parchment lined baking sheet. Heat at least 2 inches oil in a Dutch oven or skillet on medium heat. Cook patties until golden brown on each side, about 2-3 minutes. Transfer to paper towel lined plate to set. Serve warm.

Italian Omelet ⍾ *(1 serving)*

3 eggs
¼ tsp. salt
1 tbsp. unsalted butter
2 slices Prosciutto, diced

¼ cup grated mozzarella cheese
2 tbsp. chopped tomatoes
2 tbsp. chopped olives

Combine eggs and salt in a bowl and beat well with a fork. Heat a small nonstick skillet pan over medium heat, melt butter. Once the butter is melted, add eggs to skillet and immediately reduce heat to low. Using a spatula, gently pull the cooked eggs to the center, letting the liquid egg fill in the space behind it. Continue this process until the eggs are almost set. When the omelet slides around the pan easily and you can slide a spatula underneath it, flip the omelet over and remove from heat. Sprinkle cheese on top along with prosciutto, tomatoes and olives, then fold omelet over in half and transfer to plate. Serve immediately.

Lemon Blueberry Scones 🍴 *(12 drop scones)*

2 cups gluten-free all-purpose flour
½ cup granulated sugar
1 tbsp. baking powder
½ tsp. salt
½ cup butter, cut up and cold
½ cup buttermilk

1 egg, beaten
juice and zest from 1 lemon
1 cup frozen wild blueberries
½ cup confectioners sugar
1-2 tbsp. milk

Preheat oven to 400 degrees. In a food processor, combine flour, sugar, baking powder, salt, and butter. Pulse until it becomes coarse and crumbly. Transfer to a medium size mixing bowl, add buttermilk, egg, lemon juice, lemon zest, and blueberries. Stir to combine, batter will be sticky. Using a cookie scoop, drop dough onto a lined baking sheet and bake for 16-20 minutes, or until a light golden brown. Remove pan from oven, let scones cool on cooling rack. In a small mixing bowl, combine confectioners sugar and milk, stir together and drizzle on top of scones.

Lemon Poppyseed Muffins 🥄 *(12 small muffins)*

2 cups gluten-free all-purpose flour
1 tbsp. baking powder
½ tsp. salt
¾ cup granulated sugar
1 egg, beaten

2/3 cup milk
juice and zest from 1 lemon
½ cup vegetable oil
2 tbsp. poppyseeds

Preheat oven to 400 degrees. In a medium size mixing bowl, whisk together flour, baking powder, salt, and sugar. Create a well in the center. Add oil, milk, lemon juice, lemon zest, poppyseeds, and beaten egg. Stir together just until combined, batter will be lumpy. Distribute evenly into lined muffin pan, sprinkle a little more granulated sugar on top of each muffin. Place in oven to bake for 20-24 minutes, or until a light golden brown. Remove pan from oven, transfer muffins to cooling rack to cool completely.

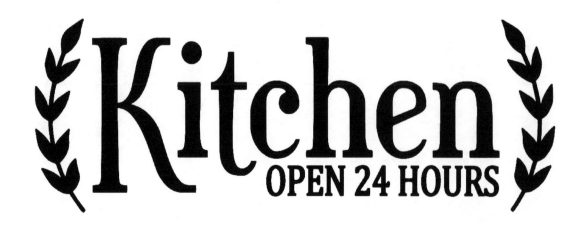

Maple Pecan Scones 🍴 *(12 drop scones)*

2 cups gluten-free all-purpose flour
½ cup light brown sugar
1 tbsp. baking powder
½ tsp. salt
½ cup butter, cut up and cold
2/3 cup buttermilk

1 egg, beaten
1 tsp. vanilla
1 tsp. maple extract
1 cup chopped pecans
½ cup confectioners sugar
3 tbsp. maple syrup

Preheat oven to 400 degrees. In a food processor, combine flour, sugar, baking powder, salt, and butter. Pulse until it becomes coarse and crumbly. Transfer to a medium size mixing bowl, add buttermilk, egg, both extracts, and chopped pecans. Stir to combine, batter will be sticky. Using a cookie scoop, drop dough onto a lined baking sheet and bake for 16-20 minutes, until a light golden brown. Remove pan from oven, let scones cool on cooling rack. In a small mixing bowl, combine confectioners sugar and maple syrup, stir together and drizzle on top of scones.

Meat Lover's Omelet 🍴 *(1 serving)*

3 eggs
¼ tsp. salt
1 tbsp. unsalted butter
¼ cup grated cheddar cheese

2 tbsp. cooked sausage crumbles
2 tbsp. diced ham
2 tbsp. real bacon bits

Combine eggs and salt in a bowl and beat well with a fork. Heat a small nonstick skillet pan over medium heat, melt butter. Once the butter is melted, add eggs to skillet and immediately reduce heat to low. Using a spatula, gently pull the cooked eggs to the center, letting the liquid egg fill in the space behind it. Continue this process until the eggs are almost set. When the omelet slides around the pan easily and you can slide a spatula underneath it, flip the omelet over and remove from heat. Sprinkle cheese on top along with sausage, ham, and bacon, then fold omelet over in half and transfer to plate. Serve immediately.

Mocha Bulletproof Coffee 🍴 *(1 serving)*

1 tbsp. coconut or MCT oil
1 tbsp. butter
¼ teaspoon cinnamon

1 scoop chocolate collagen peptides
1 scoop unflavored collagen peptides
10 oz. hot brewed coffee

Combine all ingredients in a blender or bullet and puree until smooth, serve immediately.

The fat and protein in this coffee are highly likely to keep you satisfied for hours. I love the combination of chocolate and unflavored collagen peptides for a good balance.

Morning Glory Muffins 🍴 *(12 muffins)*

½ cup raisins
2 cups gluten-free all-purpose flour
1 cup light brown sugar
1 tsp. baking soda
2 tsp. cinnamon
½ tsp. salt
2 cups grated carrots

1 large granny smith apple
½ cup shredded coconut
½ cup chopped walnuts
3 eggs
2/3 cup vegetable oil
2 tsp. vanilla
½ cup orange juice

Preheat oven to 375 degrees. Grease or line a 12-cup muffin tin with cupcake liners, set aside. Place the raisins in a small bowl and cover with hot water, set aside. In a medium size mixing bowl, combine flour, sugar, baking soda, cinnamon, and salt, whisk together well. Peel and grate the apple, add to flour mixture along with carrots, coconut, and walnuts. In a small mixing bowl, combine eggs, oil, vanilla, and orange juice, whisk together well. Pour liquid mixture into bowl with remaining ingredients, stir until combined. Drain the raisins, then stir them into the batter. Spoon batter into muffin cavities and fill almost to the top. Bake muffins for 25-28 minutes, until a toothpick inserted in center comes out clean. Remove from oven, let cool in pan for about 5 minutes before transferring to cooling racks to cool completely.

Freezing Baked Goods

At home, I keep my freezer stocked to the brim with baked goods for convenience. You can typically find muffins, scones, oatmeal bars, pancakes, waffles, etc. patiently waiting to be pulled out of the freezer to thaw and get eaten. Having a variety of items in the freezer keeps us from making terribly unhealthy or last-minute-panic-decisions about what to eat. If you're running out the door in a hurry for work, you can always grab something on the go, or stuff it in a lunch box for later.

Quiche with Grits Crust 🍴 *(14-16 servings)*

1 batch Creamy Grits
8 cups grated cheddar cheese
18 eggs
4 cups half and half

8 green onions, sliced
1 tsp. Dijon mustard
2 tsp. salt
½ tsp. black pepper

Preheat oven to 400 degrees and grease a 9x13 inch baking dish. Smooth grits evenly into the bottom of baking dish. Sprinkle cheese evenly on top of grits layer. In a large mixing bowl, beat eggs well with a whisk, add half and half, salt, pepper, and mustard, whisk again until well-combined. Pour egg mixture on top of cheese and grits. Sprinkle green onions on top. If baking immediately, bake at 400 degrees for 45 minutes or until eggs are set and cooked through.

Oatmeal (1 serving)

½ cup quick-cooking oats
1 cup water
½ tsp. ground cinnamon
½ cup frozen fruit (blueberries, etc.)

1 tbsp. chia seeds
1 tbsp. maple syrup
¼ cup chopped walnuts

In a microwave safe bowl, combine oats, water, cinnamon, and fruit. Stir together, then microwave on high for 3 - 3 ½ minutes. Remove bowl from microwave, stir in chia seeds, syrup, and nuts. Serve immediately.

This is one of my favorite go-to breakfast options for something that is quick, easy, healthy, and satisfying. This one hits all kinds of wins in my book. Hey, this is my book.

Oven Baked Bacon (4-6 servings)

½ lb. uncooked bacon

Preheat oven to 400 degrees. Line a large baking sheet with aluminum foil, place pieces of bacon side by side on foil. Bake for 12-16 minutes, depending on how crispy or tender you like your bacon. Remove baking sheet from oven, pick up bacon with tongs or a fork and set on paper towels. Lightly dab bacon with paper towels to remove extra grease, if desired. Bacon will become firm as it rests.

Pro-Tip: reserve the bacon fat for later! Pour into a glass container for storage and use fat for cooking with extra flavor.

Philly Cheese Steak Omelet (1 serving)

3 eggs
¼ tsp. salt
1 tbsp. unsalted butter
2 tbsp. diced bell peppers

1 slice provolone cheese
2 slices roast beef, diced
2 tbsp. diced onions

Combine eggs and salt in a bowl and beat well with a fork. Heat a small nonstick skillet pan over medium heat, melt butter. Once the butter is melted, add eggs to skillet and immediately reduce heat to low. Using a spatula, gently pull the cooked eggs to the center, letting the liquid egg fill in the space behind it. Continue this process until the eggs are almost set. When the omelet slides around the pan easily and you can slide a spatula underneath it, flip the omelet over and remove from heat. Lay cheese on top along with beef, peppers and onions, then fold omelet over in half and transfer to plate. Serve immediately.

Pumpkin Spice Muffins 🍴 *(10 jumbo muffins)*

2 cups gluten-free all-purpose flour
2 tsp. baking powder
1 tsp. ground cinnamon
1 tsp. pumpkin spice
1 tsp. baking soda
1 teaspoon salt
1 cup granulated sugar
2/3 cup light brown sugar

4 eggs
15 oz. can pumpkin puree
1 cup vegetable oil
1 tsp. vanilla
½ cup gluten-free all-purpose flour
½ cup light brown sugar
½ tsp. cinnamon
¼ cup butter, melted

Preheat oven to 450 degrees. In a standing mixer or medium size mixing bowl, combine flour, baking powder, cinnamon, pumpkin spice, baking soda, salt, sugars, eggs, pumpkin, oil, and vanilla. Beat with electric mixer at medium speed for 1-2 minutes, until well-combined. Line 2 jumbo muffin pans with liners, distribute batter evenly into cavities, about 2/3 full. In a small mixing bowl, combine ½ cup light brown sugar, ½ cup flour, cinnamon, and melted butter. Toss together until combined, then sprinkle evenly over each muffin. Place pans in oven and bake for 12 minutes. Reduce oven temperature to 350 degrees, continue baking for another 16-18 minutes, or until toothpick inserted in muffins comes out clean. Remove pans from oven and let cool for about 5 minutes before removing muffins from pans and cooling completely on cooling racks. Serve immediately or wrap individually in plastic wrap and store in freezer.

Pumpkin Donuts 🍴 *(12 donuts)*

1 ½ cups gluten-free all-purpose flour
½ cup light brown sugar
½ tbsp. baking powder
1 tsp. cinnamon
½ tsp. salt
¼ tsp. baking soda

1 cup pureed pumpkin
2 eggs
¼ cup butter, softened
¼ cup milk
1 cup confectioners sugar
2-3 tbsp. milk

Preheat oven to 325 degrees, grease two donut pans with cooking spray and set aside. In a medium size mixing bowl, combine flour, sugar, baking powder, cinnamon, salt and baking soda, whisk together. Add pumpkin, eggs, milk and butter. Using an electric mixer, beat at medium speed for about 1 minute, just until well combined. Spoon batter into a large pastry bag, cut about 1 inch off the tip of the pastry bag. Pipe batter into donut pan, then place in oven and bake for 8-10 minutes (or until donut springs back lightly when touched). Remove from oven and turn donuts out of pan onto a parchment paper lined cookie sheet. Stir together confectioners sugar and 2-3 tablespoons milk. Dip each donut in glaze, return to parchment paper to cool and set. Best served immediately.

Pumpkin Oatmeal Bars 🍴 *(16 bars)*

15 oz. can pumpkin puree
1 ½ cups oat milk
1 ½ cups maple syrup
1 tbsp. vanilla

1 tbsp. cinnamon
5 cups rolled oats
1 cup pumpkin seeds

Preheat oven to 350 degrees. In a medium size mixing bowl, combine pumpkin, maple syrup, and cinnamon. Whisk together well. Add rolled oats and stir together until well-combined. Spoon into a 9x13 inch pan that has been lined with parchment paper and press into an even layer. Sprinkle pumpkin seeds on top and bake for 35-40 minutes. Remove pan from oven and cool completely before cutting into bars. Wrap individually in plastic wrap and store in refrigerator for up to 5 days, or in the freezer for 6 months.

Red Velvet Donuts 🍴 *(12 donuts)*

5 tbsp. butter, softened
½ cup granulated sugar
1 ½ cups gluten-free all-purpose flour
2 tsp. baking powder
¼ tsp. salt
2 tsp. unsweetened cocoa

½ tsp. vinegar
1 egg
½ cup buttermilk
½ tbsp. red food coloring
1 cup confectioners sugar
2-3 tsp. milk

Preheat oven to 350 degrees. Cream the butter and sugar until well blended, add eggs. Continue mixing, then add remaining ingredients and beat well at medium speed. Dough will be thick. Spoon into zipper freezer bag or cake decorating bag. Spray donut pan with cooking spray that has flour, or grease and flour pan. Pipe dough into pan, filling about 2/3 of the way full. Bake for 15 minutes, cool completely. Stir together confectioners sugar and milk. Dunk each donut in glaze, let set on wire rack.

Red Velvet Waffles 🍴 *(4 large waffles)*

2 cups gluten-free baking mix
1 tbsp. unsweetened cocoa
1 1/3 cups milk
2 tbsp. white vinegar

2 tbsp. vegetable oil
1 egg, beaten
Red food coloring

Heat a waffle maker and coat plates with cooking spray. In a medium mixing bowl, whisk together all ingredients to make waffle batter. When waffle maker indicates it's ready, pour ¾ cup batter in center of plates, and close. Open waffle maker and use a fork to remove from plates. Serve warm and drizzle with maple syrup.

Pro-Tip: the amount of food coloring depends on if you're using liquid or paste. You'll need less with paste, more with liquid.

Sausage Gravy (4-6 servings)

1 lb. ground pork sausage
2 tbsp. butter
1/3 cup gluten-free all-purpose flour (no XG)
3 cups half and half

¼ tsp. garlic powder
¼ tsp. onion powder
¼ tsp. salt
¼ tsp. black pepper

Cook the sausage in a large skillet over medium heat until browned and no longer pink. Add butter, stir until melted. Sprinkle flour into pan over sausage and butter, stir and continue to cook for another 2 minutes. Pour half and half into the pan slowly, stirring constantly until smooth. Add seasonings and stir, adjust seasoning if needed. Sauce will thicken as is continues to cook. Serve warm over biscuits.

Pro-Tip: to make this dairy-free, use plant butter and 1–1 ½ cups non-dairy milk. Non-dairy milk is typically thinner than half and half, which is why you will need less for this conversion. If you want to make this Low-Carb, omit the flour and use 1 tsp. xanthan gum as a thickening agent.

Shirred Eggs with Ham (4 servings)

¼ cup butter, softened
¼ lb. thinly sliced deli ham
8 eggs

salt and pepper (to taste)
¼ cup heavy cream
¼ cup grated parmesan cheese

Preheat oven to 325 degrees. Rub 1 tablespoon butter into each of four 6 oz. ramekin dishes, set dishes on a baking pan. Place slices of ham into each dish on top of butter. Break two eggs into each ramekin on top of ham, sprinkle with salt and pepper. Bake until the eggs begin to set, about 8-10 minutes. Remove pan from oven, pour 1 tablespoon heavy cream into each ramekin, followed by 1 tablespoon parmesan cheese. Return to oven and bake for another 3-5 minutes. Serve warm.

Slow Cooker Breakfast Casserole (6-8 servings)

12 eggs, beaten
2 cups milk
32 oz. frozen diced hashbrown potatoes

4.5 oz. package real bacon bits
3 cups grated sharp cheddar cheese
Salt and pepper to taste

In a medium mixing bowl, whisk together eggs, milk, and desired salt and pepper, set aside. Coat a 4-quart slow cooker with cooking spray. Pour half of hashbrowns into an even layer in slow cooker, followed by half of bacon bits, and 1 ½ cups cheddar. Repeat layering. Pour liquid ingredients on top of potatoes, bacon, and cheese. Set slow cooker on low, cover, and let cook for approximately 8-10 hours.

Southwest Omelet ♀ (*1 serving*)

3 eggs	¼ cup grated pepper jack cheese
¼ tsp. salt	¼ cup pico de gallo
1 tbsp. unsalted butter	½ avocado, pitted and sliced

Combine eggs and salt in a bowl and beat well with a fork. Heat a small nonstick skillet pan over medium heat, melt butter. Once the butter is melted, add eggs to skillet and immediately reduce heat to low. Using a spatula, gently pull the cooked eggs to the center, letting the liquid egg fill in the space behind it. Continue this process until the eggs are almost set. When the omelet slides around the pan easily and you can slide a spatula underneath it, flip the omelet over and remove from heat. Sprinkle cheese on top along with pico de gallo, then fold omelet over in half and transfer to plate. Serve with sliced avocado on top.

Steak and Eggs ♀ (*2-4 servings*)

6 oz. leftover cooked steak	2 tbsp. unsalted butter
6 eggs	¼ tsp. salt

Break eggs into a bowl and whisk together well with a fork. Heat a nonstick skillet pan on medium heat and add butter. When butter has melted, pour in eggs and reduce heat to low/medium. Using a spatula, gently stir eggs as they cook. Add steak and sprinkle in salt, continue stirring and cooking until eggs are cooked through and steak is hot. Serve immediately.

♀**Pro-Tip:** use leftover steak from a grilled steak at home or from a restaurant. Store in refrigerator, then slice into bite-size pieces just before preparing eggs.

I don't drink coffee to wake up. I wake up to drink coffee.

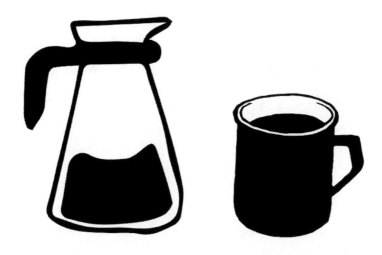

Sticky Buns ♟♟♟ *(12 rolls)*

½ cup granulated sugar
1 cup milk (110-115 degrees)
1 tbsp. instant/rapid yeast
¼ cup unsalted butter, melted and cooled
2 large eggs, room temperature
1 tsp. apple cider vinegar
3 ¼ cups gluten-free all-purpose flour

2 tsp. baking powder
½ tsp. salt
½ cup half and half
¼ cup unsalted butter, softened
1 cup light brown sugar
2 tbsp. cinnamon
½ cup chopped pecans

Preheat oven to 350 degrees. In a standing mixer, combine granulated sugar, warmed milk, and yeast. Cover with a kitchen towel and let it bubble up for about 2-3 minutes. Beat eggs in a small bowl before adding to large mixing bowl along with melted butter and apple cider vinegar. Add flour, baking powder, and salt to bowl. Using paddle attachment, mix for 1-2 minutes, until fully combined. Change paddle attachment to dough hook, mix on medium speed for 3-5 minutes. Transfer dough to a greased glass or metal bowl. Wet hands with warm water, rub the dough to make it smooth. Cover bowl with plastic wrap and set inside a larger bowl. Pour hot water inside larger bowl, surrounding the bowl with dough (this helps it rise). Cover both bowls with a kitchen towel and let rise for 20 minutes. In a small bowl, toss together light brown sugar and cinnamon, set aside. Lay a large piece of parchment paper on flat surface and grease with cooking spray. Place dough on top, sprinkle with extra gluten-free flour or rice flour, roll out dough using a rolling pin to ½ inch thick and into a 12x14 inch rectangle. Spread softened butter evenly on top, then sprinkle brown sugar cinnamon mixture over butter along with chopped pecans and press down. Use the edge of the parchment paper to fold the longest end up to start the roll. Roll the dough up tightly to form a log. Cut the log in half, then cut each half into six rolls using dental floss. Grease a 9x13 inch baking dish with cooking spray, then place the rolls inside. Pour caramel sauce on top of rolls and bake for 20-25 minutes, until a light golden brown. Cool slightly and serve.

Caramel Sauce Topping ♟

½ cup butter
1 cup dark brown sugar
¼ tsp. salt

¼ cup heavy cream
1 cup chopped pecans

Combine butter and dark brown sugar in a small saucepan on medium heat. Cook until sugar dissolves, add heavy cream and salt, mix well but do not let boil. Pour over rolls before baking and sprinkle with chopped pecans.

Strawberry Pound Cake French Toast ♐ *(4 servings)*

2 large eggs
1 cup half and half
Pinch of salt
1 tbsp. granulated sugar

1 tsp. vanilla
1 tsp. cinnamon
1 loaf Pound Cake (p. 223)
1-pint fresh strawberries, sliced

In a medium size mixing bowl, whisk together eggs, half and half, salt, sugar, vanilla, and ground cinnamon. Heat a large non-stick skillet or griddle on medium heat. Slice Pound Cake into thick pieces (about 1 inch thick). Dip each piece of bread into mixture and coat both sides before placing on griddle. Cook until golden brown on each side, about 2-3 minutes. Serve with fresh strawberries and Strawberry Maple Syrup.

Strawberry Maple Syrup ♐ (4-6 servings)

2 cups frozen strawberries, thawed*   ½ cup maple syrup

Combine both ingredients in a blender and puree until smooth. Pour through a fine mesh strainer and store in refrigerator for up to 2 weeks.

Pro-Tip: switch up the fruit by using blueberries or raspberries for other pancakes, waffles, and French toast!

Sweet Potato Pancakes ♐ (6-8 servings)

2 cups gluten-free all-purpose flour
¼ cup light brown sugar
2 tsp. baking powder
1 tsp. baking soda
1 tsp. cinnamon
½ tsp. salt

1 ¾ cups buttermilk
1 cup canned sweet potatoes (yams)
1 egg
1 tsp. vanilla
2 tbsp. butter, melted

In a medium size mixing bowl, combine flour, sugar, baking powder, baking soda, cinnamon, and salt. Whisk together and set aside. In a blender, combine buttermilk, sweet potatoes, egg, vanilla, and melted butter. Puree until smooth, pour into mixing bowl with dry ingredients and whisk together until well combined. Heat a large skillet over medium heat, and coat with cooking spray. Pour ¼ cupfuls of batter onto the skillet and cook until bubbles appear on the surface. Flip with a flexible spatula and cook until lightly browned on the other side. Serve warm with butter and maple syrup.

Pro-Tip: these can also be made as **Pumpkin Pancakes**, just switch out the sweet potatoes for canned pumpkin!

Tiramisu Pancake Stack 🍴 *(3-5 servings)*

9-10 gluten-free pancakes
1 cup coffee, cooled
8 oz. mascarpone cheese

8 oz. frozen whipped topping, thawed
2 tbsp. confectioners sugar
gluten-free chocolate syrup or ganache

Prepare pancakes as desired, let cool slightly. In a medium size mixing bowl, combine mascarpone cheese, whipped topping, and confectioners sugar. Beat at medium speed with electric mixer for about 1 minute, set aside. Place a cooled pancake on plate. Brush pancake with 1 tablespoon coffee, then spoon ¼ cup cream mixture on top of pancake and spread into an even layer. Place another cooled pancake on top, repeating coffee and cream process one or two more times, depending on how many layers of pancakes you desire. Drizzle with chocolate syrup and serve immediately.

🍴**Pro-Tip:** pancakes can be made fresh or for convenience use frozen gluten-free pancakes!

Veggie Scramble 🍴 *(1 serving)*

1 tbsp. coconut oil
1 clove garlic, minced
¼ cup diced onion
¼ cup diced bell pepper

2 eggs
½ cup egg whites
½ avocado
salt and pepper to taste

Heat oil in a small skillet pan on medium heat, add diced veggies and sauté until tender. Combine eggs and egg whites in a bowl and beat with a fork or whisk. Pour eggs into pan and reduce heat to low/medium, stirring occasionally and cook until eggs are cooked through. Sprinkle with salt and pepper, spoon eggs onto a plate. Remove pit from avocado and scoop out of peel, dice and serve on top of eggs.

Waffles 🍴 *(4-6 waffles)*

1 1/3 cups gluten-free all-purpose flour
4 tsp. baking powder
½ tsp. salt
1 tbsp. sugar

2 eggs, separated
½ cup butter, melted
1 tsp. vanilla
1 ¾ cups milk

In a large mixing bowl, whisk together all dry ingredients. Separate the eggs, adding the yolks to the dry ingredient mixture, and placing the whites in a small mixing bowl. Beat whites at medium speed with electric mixer until white and soft peaks form, set aside. Add milk, melted butter and vanilla to dry ingredient mixture, whisk together well. Gently fold stiff egg whites into mixture. Pour batter into hot waffle iron and bake until golden brown. Serve warm with maple syrup or other fruit syrup.

Western Omelet *(1 serving)*

3 eggs
¼ tsp. salt
1 tbsp. unsalted butter
2 tbsp. diced bell peppers

¼ cup grated cheddar cheese
2 tbsp. diced ham
2 tbsp. diced onions

Combine eggs and salt in a bowl and beat well with a fork. Heat a small nonstick skillet pan over medium heat, melt butter. Once the butter is melted, add eggs to skillet and immediately reduce heat to low. Using a spatula, gently pull the cooked eggs to the center, letting the liquid egg fill in the space behind it. Continue this process until the eggs are almost set. When the omelet slides around the pan easily and you can slide a spatula underneath it, flip the omelet over and remove from heat. Lay cheese on top along with ham, peppers and onions, then fold omelet over in half and transfer to plate. Serve immediately.

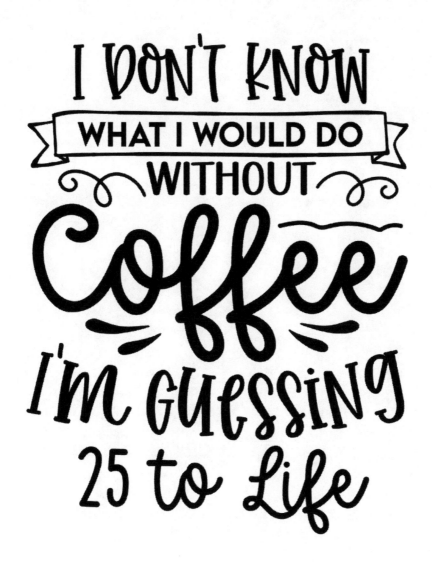

Soups, Sauces & Salads

Beer Cheddar Soup ₰ *(6-8 servings)*

1 cup unsalted butter
1 onion, diced
1 red bell pepper, diced
2 cloves garlic, minced
½ cup gluten-free all-purpose flour (no XG)
12 oz. gluten-free light beer
3 cups chicken broth

2 cups half and half
2 lbs. grated cheddar cheese
24 oz. bag frozen steam-n-mash potatoes
1 lb. smoked sausage link, diced
½ tsp. paprika
2 tsp. salt

Melt butter in stock pot on medium heat, add onions and bell peppers. Cook until vegetables are soft, add garlic, then whisk in flour and continue cooking for 1 minute. Add beer and whisk again, it will thicken quickly. Slowly whisk in chicken broth, puree soup using an immersion blender, or transfer soup to blender and puree. Cook potatoes according to package directions, mash with a potato masher in a medium size mixing bowl and set aside. Add half and half, paprika, and salt to stock pot and stir together, continue cooking. Add grated cheese and stir until cheese is completely melted. Stir in mashed potatoes and diced sausage, cook for another 2-3 minutes and serve hot.

₰ Pro-Tip: if your grocery store doesn't carry steam-n-mash potatoes, improvise! Take 3-4 medium size russet potatoes, price all over with a fork and lightly rub with olive oil. Bake in a 350-degree oven for about 1 hour, until potatoes are soft. Slice open potatoes, scoop out pulp and use in the soup recipe.

Black Bean Tortilla Soup ₰ *(6-8 servings)*

½ onion, diced
3 cloves garlic, minced
¼ cup olive oil
1 poblano pepper
1 corn tortilla
12 oz. frozen corn, thawed

2 (15 oz). cans black beans
15 oz. can pinto beans
8 oz. can tomato sauce
4 cups vegetable broth
2-3 tsp. salt
1 tsp. black pepper

Heat olive oil in large pot on medium heat. Add onion, poblano peppers and garlic, sauté until vegetables are tender. Tear corn tortillas into pieces, add to pot and continue to cook for another 1-2 minutes. Add two cups of the vegetable broth, simmer for about five minutes. Remove from heat to cool slightly, pour veggies into blender and puree until smooth (or use an immersion blender and puree directly in the pot). Transfer back to pot, add remaining vegetable broth, tomato sauce, and corn, stir well and cook for about 5 more minutes. Rinse and drain beans, add to soup continue cooking until corn is tender and soup is thoroughly heated through. Add salt and pepper, stir well and serve hot.

This is basically the vegan or plant-based version of Chicken Tortilla Soup. I included both recipes in this book because I make both versions on a semi-regular basis!

Chicken Pot Pie Soup 🥄 *(6-8 servings)*

1 lb. butter
1 cup gluten-free all-purpose flour (no XG)
2 tbsp. onion powder
4 cups chicken broth
2 cups whole milk

2 lbs. cooked chicken, diced
1 lb. frozen mixed veggies, thawed
1 tsp. salt
¼ tsp. black pepper

Melt butter in large pot on medium heat. When butter is melted, whisk in flour and onion powder, cook for 1 minute. Slowly whisk in chicken broth and milk, continue cooking for about 10 minutes, stirring occasionally until soup thickens. Stir in chicken, veggies, salt, and pepper, cook for another 5 minutes. Serve hot.

Chicken Tortilla Soup 🥄 *(6-8 servings)*

½ onion, diced
3 cloves garlic, minced
¼ cup olive oil
1 poblano pepper
1 corn tortilla
12 oz. frozen corn, thawed

15 oz. can black beans
1 lb. cooked chicken, diced
8 oz. can tomato sauce
4 cups chicken broth
2-3 tsp. salt
1 tsp. black pepper

Heat olive oil in large pot on medium heat. Add onion, poblano peppers and garlic; sauté until vegetables are tender. Add corn tortillas and continue to cook for another 1-2 minutes. Add two cups of the chicken broth, simmer for about five minutes. Remove from heat to cool slightly, pour veggies into blender and puree until smooth (or use an immersion blender and puree directly in the pot). Transfer back to pot, add remaining chicken broth, tomato sauce, and corn, stir well and cook for about 5 more minutes. Add black beans and chicken, continue cooking until corn is tender and soup is thoroughly heated through. Add salt and pepper, stir well and serve hot.

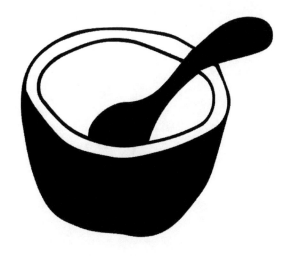

Corn Chowder 🥄 *(6-8 servings)*

½ cup butter
¼ cup gluten-free all-purpose flour (no XG)
½ onion, diced
1 medium size russet potato
4 cups chicken broth
2 cups heavy cream

8 oz. package diced ham
24 oz. frozen corn, thawed
½ cup grated parmesan
1 tsp. salt
½ tsp. black pepper
2 tsp. dried basil

Melt the butter in a large pot over medium heat. Add onion, cook until soft. Stir in the flour and cook for about 1-2 minutes. Slowly whisk in the chicken broth, making sure everything dissolves together. Add potatoes, stir occasionally and cook for 15-20 minutes (or until potatoes are tender). When potatoes are done cooking, add heavy cream, corn, and ham. Cook until heated through, add parmesan, salt, basil, and pepper. Continue cooking until cheese is melted and soup is hot. Serve and garnish with freshly grated cheddar, bacon bits, and green onions if desired.

Cream of Broccoli Soup 🥄 *(6-8 servings)*

¼ cup butter
½ onion, diced
2 tbsp. gluten-free all-purpose flour (no XG)
20 oz. frozen chopped broccoli, thawed
3 cups chicken broth

1 cup heavy cream
1-2 tsp. salt
¼ tsp. black pepper
½ cup grated parmesan
1 lb. grated sharp cheddar cheese

Melt butter in a large pot over medium heat. Add onion, cook until soft. Stir in the flour and cook for about 1 minute. Slowly whisk in the chicken broth, making sure everything dissolves together. Add broccoli and cook for about 10 minutes. Add heavy cream, salt, and pepper. Puree soup with immersion blender for a smoother consistency, but you can omit this step for a chunkier soup. Add parmesan and cheddar cheeses, remove pot from heat and stir until cheeses are melted, serve hot.

Easy Chili 🥄 *(6-8 servings)*

1 lb. ground beef
1 tbsp. onion powder
1 tbsp. light brown sugar

1 tbsp. chili powder
28 oz. gluten-free baked beans
15 oz. tomato sauce

In a large pot on medium heat, cook ground beef until browned, drain excess liquid. Add onion powder, brown sugar, and chili powder, stir. Add remaining ingredients and stir again, continue to cook on low/medium heat until heated through. Serve hot, goes well with cornbread!

French Onion Soup 🍴 *(6-8 servings)*

½ cup butter
2 onions, sliced
2 cloves garlic, minced
2 tsp. granulated sugar
1 tsp. salt
½ tsp. black pepper

4 cups beef broth
½ cup white wine
2 cups water
1 tsp. dried thyme
2 bay leaves
1 cup grated gruyere cheese

In a large pot on medium heat, melt butter. Add onions, cover and cook until tender, about 5 minutes. Add garlic, sugar, salt, and pepper, cover and reduce heat to low for 30 minutes until the onions are caramelized, stirring occasionally. Add broth, wine, water, thyme, and bay leaves. Cover and simmer on low for another hour. Transfer soup to bowls, top each bowl with gluten-free bread (if desired) followed by gruyere cheese. Place bowls on a pan and put under broiler in oven until cheese is melted. Serve immediately.

Gumbo 🍴 *(6-8 servings)*

1 cup gluten-free all-purpose flour (no XG)
2/3 cup oil
6 cups chicken broth
1 yellow onion, diced
1 green bell pepper, seeded and diced
4 stalks celery, diced
1 bunch green onion, finely chopped

1 bunch chopped fresh parsley
3 cloves garlic, minced
2 tbsp. Cajun seasoning
12 oz. package andouille sausage, sliced
1 lb. cooked chicken, diced
24 oz. frozen cooked shrimp, thawed

Combine flour and oil in a large stock pot on low/medium heat, stirring constantly for 30-45 minutes. When done cooking, it should be a dark brown color and have a soft consistency. Add chicken broth, 2 cups at a time, whisking to prevent clumps. Add onion, bell pepper, celery, green onion, parsley, and garlic. Bring to a boil and cook for 8-10 minutes, or until vegetables are slightly tender. Add Cajun seasoning, sausage, chicken, and shrimp. Continue cooking until meat is hot, add salt to taste if needed. Serve warm over rice, store any leftovers in refrigerator for up to 7 days.

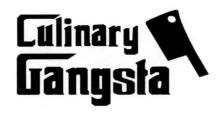

Ham Chowder *(6-8 servings)*

½ cup butter
1 onion, diced
2 carrots, diced
½ cup gluten-free all-purpose flour (no XG)
3 cups milk

3 cups chicken broth
1 potato, peeled and diced
16 oz. diced ham
½ cup real bacon bits
Salt and pepper to taste

Heat butter in a large pot on medium heat. When melted, add onion and carrots, cook until tender. Add flour, stir well. Slowly add milk then chicken broth, stirring to prevent clumps. Add potato, continue to cook for about 10-12 minutes or until potatoes are tender. Stir in ham and bacon, season with salt and pepper to taste.

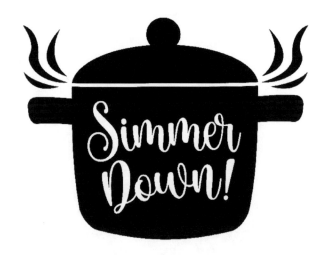

Hearty Vegetable Chowder *(6-8 servings)*

1 onion, diced
4 stalks celery, diced
¼ cup olive oil
2 lbs. steam-in-a-bag cauliflower
2 cups water, divided

¼ cup butter
4 cups vegetable broth
2 lbs. frozen mixed veggies, thawed
2-3 tsp. salt
½ tsp. black pepper

Place onion, celery, and oil in a large pot on medium heat on the stove. While vegetables are cooking, stir occasionally and cook each bag of cauliflower in microwave according to package instructions. Pour 1 cup water in a blender, then add 1 bag cooked cauliflower and puree until smooth. Add butter and the remaining bag of cauliflower, pureeing again until smooth. Pour pureed cauliflower, vegetable broth, and remaining 1 cup water into the pot and stir well. Add mixed vegetables, salt and pepper, cover and continue cooking for about 10 minutes. Serve hot.

Hillbilly Chili Ⓘ *(6-8 servings)*

1 lb. ground sausage

16 oz. jar Pace's® restaurant style salsa

28 oz. gluten-free baked beans

Cook sausage on medium heat in a large pot until browned and completely cooked through, drain and return to pot. Add salsa and baked beans, stir and cook until hot and serve warm.

Pro-Tip: this recipe is versatile and can be served as a chili or as a dip. If you make this as a dip, transfer to a slow cooker on warm setting and serve with tortilla chips.

Leftover Turkey Chowder Ⓘ *(6-8 servings)*

½ cup butter

1 onion, diced

4 stalks celery, diced

3 medium carrots, peeled and grated

2 cloves garlic, minced

2 radishes, peeled and chopped

3 parsnips, peeled and grated

32 oz. chicken bone broth

32 oz. water

2-3 tsp. sea salt

1 tsp. black pepper

2-3 lbs. cooked turkey

1 lb. frozen corn, thawed

Melt butter in a large pot on medium heat. Add onion and celery, cook until tender. Add carrots, garlic, radishes, parsnips, bone broth and water. Bring to a boil and cook until vegetables are tender, about 10-15 minutes. Using an immersion blender, puree soup to a smooth, chowder-like consistency. Add salt and pepper, tear cooked turkey into bite-size pieces before adding to soup. Stir in corn and cook until heated through, serve warm.

Lentil Soup Ⓘ *(6-8 servings)*

¼ cup olive oil

1 medium onion, diced

2 carrots, peeled and diced

4 garlic cloves, minced

2 tsp. ground cumin

1 tsp. curry powder

½ tsp. dried thyme

28 oz. can diced tomatoes, drained

1 cup brown lentils, rinsed

4 cups vegetable broth

2 cups water

salt and pepper to taste

Heat olive oil in a large pot on medium heat. Add onion and carrot, cook and stir often until onion has softened, about 5 minutes. Add garlic, cumin, curry, and dried thyme. Stir constantly and cook until fragrant, about 30 seconds. Add diced tomatoes and stir, cook for another couple minutes. Add lentils, broth, water, and season with salt and pepper. Increase heat and bring soup to a boil, then partially cover and reduce heat to a simmer for 25-30 minutes or until lentils are tender but still hold their shape. Use an immersion blender to partially blend the soup. Serve hot.

Loaded Baked Potato Soup 🥄 *(6-8 servings)*

2 (24 oz.) packages frozen steam 'n mash potatoes
½ cup unsalted butter
½ onion, diced
2 cloves garlic, minced
¼ cup gluten-free all-purpose flour (no XG)

4 cups chicken broth
2 cups heavy cream
1-2 tsp. salt
1 tsp. black pepper
1 cup grated cheddar cheese

Cook potatoes according to package directions, mash with a potato masher in a medium size mixing bowl and set aside. Melt butter in large pot on medium heat, add diced onion. Cook until onions are soft, add garlic, then stir in flour and continue cooking for 1 minute. Stir in chicken broth. Puree soup using an immersion blender (or transfer soup to blender and puree). Add heavy cream, salt, and pepper to pot and stir together, continue cooking. Stir in mashed potatoes and cheese, cook for another 2-3 minutes until cheese is melted. Serve hot, garnish with bacon bits, sour cream and green onions if desired.

Minestrone 🍴 *(6-8 servings)*

¼ cup olive oil
1 yellow onion, diced
2 carrots, peeled and diced
2 stalks celery, chopped
¼ cup tomato paste
1 medium zucchini, diced
1 cup frozen cut green beans, thawed
4 cloves garlic, minced
½ tsp. dried oregano
½ tsp. dried thyme

28 oz. can diced tomatoes
4 cups vegetable broth
2 cups water
1 tsp. salt
2 bay leaves
¼ tsp. black pepper
1 cup gluten-free pasta
15 oz. can Great Northern beans
grated parmesan cheese (optional)

Heat olive oil in a large pot on medium heat. When the oil is hot, add onion, carrots, celery, and tomato paste. Cook until the vegetables are tender, stirring often. Add zucchini, green beans, garlic, oregano, and thyme. Continue to cook for another 2 minutes, stirring frequently. Add the can of diced tomatoes and their juices, along with vegetable broth and water. Add salt, bay leaves, and black pepper. Increase heat to medium/high to bring soup to a boil, then partially cover pot with lid and cook for 15 minutes. Rinse and drain beans, add to pot along with pasta and cook uncovered for another 20 minutes or until pasta is al dente. Remove pot from heat, then remove bay leaves. Season with more salt and pepper, if desired. Serve warm with a sprinkle of parmesan cheese.

Pro-Tip: for a gluten-free pasta in this recipe, I typically like to use a smaller type of pasta, such as elbows. They're easy to scoop up in a spoon but remember there are certain types of pasta that won't hold up as well. For this recipe, I prefer to use Ronzoni brand elbow pasta.

New England Clam Chowder 🍴 *(6-8 servings)*

3 (6.5 oz.) cans minced clams
1 cup clam juice
¼ cup butter
2 stalks celery, diced
1 onion, diced
1 lb. russet potatoes (peeled and diced)
4 cloves garlic, minced
1/3 cup gluten-free all-purpose flour (no XG)

2 cups chicken broth
2 bay leaves
8 oz. diced ham
½ tsp. dried parsley
½ tsp. dried oregano
½ tsp. salt
¼ tsp. black pepper
1 cup heavy cream

Drain juice from clam cans into a measuring cup, add more from bottle to equal about 2 ½ cups and set aside. In a large pot on medium heat, melt butter. Add diced celery and onion, cook for 6-8 minutes or until onions are tender. Add potatoes and garlic, sauté for about 30 seconds. Add flour and cook for another 60 seconds. Stir in broth, clam juice, bay leaves, and all other seasonings. Bring to a boil, then reduce to a simmer and cook for 15-20 minutes or until potatoes are tender. Remove bay leaves, add heavy cream and stir. Remove from heat, stir in clams and diced ham, adjust salt and pepper as needed and cook until meats are hot. Serve warm.

Pizza Soup 🍴 *(6-8 servings)*

¼ cup olive oil
1 onion, diced
1 green bell pepper, seeded and diced
8 oz. white button mushrooms, diced
3 cloves garlic, minced
1 tsp. sea salt

28 oz. can crushed tomatoes
1 tbsp. Italian seasoning
32 oz. vegetable broth
1 lb. smoked sausage, diced
5 oz. uncured pepperoni, quartered
½ cup grated parmesan cheese
1 cup grated mozzarella cheese

Heat oil in a large pot on medium heat. Add onion, bell pepper, and mushrooms. Cook, stirring occasionally, until vegetables are tender, about 5-6 minutes. Add garlic, cook for one more minute before adding salt, crushed tomatoes, Italian seasoning, and vegetable broth. Continue cooking for another 5 minutes, add sausage and pepperoni. Cook for another 5-10 minutes, until soup is hot. Transfer to bowls, garnish with grated parmesan and mozzarella cheeses.

Pro-Tip: this is a Low-Carb recipe, and a great side dish would be any sort of bread used with Fathead Dough (p. 218), like rolls or breadsticks. If you're not into Low-Carb but do want some breadsticks, check out the Garlic Breadsticks recipe on p. 218!

Roasted Vegetable Soup ♈ *(6-8 servings)*

½ cup olive oil, divided
4 stalks celery, diced
3 cloves garlic, minced
1 onion, diced
4 cups vegetable broth
29 oz. can tomato sauce
2 medium zucchini

2 medium squash
6 oz. mushrooms
3 carrots, peeled and diced
1 potato, peeled and diced
12 oz. frozen corn, thawed
2-3 tsp. salt
1 tsp. black pepper

Preheat oven to 375 degrees. Heat ¼ cup olive oil on medium heat in a large pot. When oil is hot, add celery and onion. Cook for 4-5 minutes, until onion is tender. Add garlic, cook for about 1 minute until fragrant. Stir in vegetable broth and tomato sauce. Cut zucchini and squash into 1-inch chunks and place in a medium size mixing bowl. Wipe mushrooms using a damp paper towel and remove stems, then chop in half and add to bowl with zucchini and squash. Add remaining ¼ cup olive oil and toss to coat well, then spread into a greased 9x13 inch baking dish and roast veggies in oven for 20 minutes or until tender. Add diced carrots and potatoes to pot while veggies are roasting in oven, cooking for about 15 minutes or until tender. When veggies are done roasting, spoon into stock pot along with corn, salt, and black pepper. Adjust seasonings as needed, serve warm.

Shrimp Bisque ♈ *(6-8 servings)*

½ cup butter
1 onion, diced
3 cloves garlic, minced
½ cup white wine or cooking sherry
2 (28 oz.) cans crushed tomatoes
29 oz. tomato sauce

2 cups seafood stock
12 oz. frozen cooked shrimp, thawed
2 tsp. dried basil
1 tsp. dried oregano
1-2 tsp. salt
½ cup grated parmesan

Melt butter in a pot on medium heat. Add diced onion and cook until tender. Add garlic and stir, continue cooking for one minute. Pour in cooking sherry and cook for another minute, then add crushed tomatoes, tomato sauce, seafood stock, shrimp, basil, oregano, and salt. Continue cooking for about 8-10 minutes. Using an immersion blender, puree soup until smooth. Add parmesan cheese and continue cooking for another 2-3 minutes, until cheese has melted. Serve hot.

The first time I had Shrimp Bisque was when I was working in a restaurant that served Pita Points (p. 32). You would have thought I had discovered Wonderland when I dipped a Pita Point into this bisque, and I still envision myself with my eyes closed and a goofy grin on my face was enjoying this combination a little too much.

Split Pea Soup ♈ *(6-8 servings)*

2 ¼ cups dried split peas
4 cups water
4 cups chicken bone broth
2 onions, diced
½ tsp. salt

¼ tsp. black pepper
3 stalks celery, diced
3 carrots, peeled and diced
1 potato, peeled and diced
8 oz. diced ham

Let peas soak in water overnight in a large pot. Drain and rinse peas before returning to pot. Add water, bone broth, onions, salt, and pepper to pot, cover and bring to a boil. Reduce heat and simmer for 1 ½ hours, stirring occasionally. Add celery, carrots, and potatoes. Cook for another 30-40 minutes, until vegetables are tender. Add ham and stir, continue cooking for another 2-3 minutes before serving.

Sweet Potato Soup ♈ *(6-8 servings)*

2 tbsp. olive oil
1 medium yellow onion, chopped
2 stalks celery, diced
3 medium sweet potatoes, peeled and cubed
3 cloves garlic, minced
½ tsp. dried oregano

½ tsp. ginger
½ tsp. smoked paprika
salt and pepper to taste
3 cups vegetable broth
14 oz. can full-fat coconut milk

Heat oil in a large pot over medium heat. Add onion and celery, sauté until soft, about 5-6 minutes. Add sweet potatoes, cook until they begin to soften, about 10 minutes. Stir in garlic, oregano, ginger, paprika, salt and pepper. Add vegetable broth and coconut milk, bring to a boil, cover, and reduce heat to a simmer. Cook for about 20-30 minutes, or until potatoes are tender. Using an immersion blender, puree soup until smooth. If soup is too thick, add more broth or water. Serve hot and garnish with sour cream, if desired.

Tomato Bisque ♈ *(6-8 servings)*

½ cup butter
1 onion, diced
3 cloves garlic, minced
½ cup white wine or cooking sherry
2 (28 oz.) cans crushed tomatoes
29 oz. tomato sauce

2 cups heavy cream
½ cup grated parmesan
2 tsp. dried basil
1 tsp. dried oregano
1-2 tsp. salt
1 tbsp. granulated sugar

Melt butter in a large pot on medium heat. Add diced onion and cook until tender. Add garlic and stir, continue cooking for one minute. Pour in cooking sherry and cook for another minute, then add crushed tomatoes, tomato sauce, heavy cream, basil, oregano, salt, and sugar. Continue cooking for about 8-10 minutes. Using an immersion blender, puree soup until smooth. Add parmesan cheese and continue cooking for another 2-3 minutes, until cheese has melted. Serve hot.

Vegetable Beef Soup *(6-8 servings)*

1 lb. lean ground beef
1 medium onion, diced
2 cloves garlic, minced
1 tsp. Italian seasoning
6 cups beef broth

15 oz. can diced tomatoes, drained
1 medium potato, peeled and cubed
1 lb. frozen mixed veggies*
Salt and pepper to taste

Cook ground beef on medium heat in a large pot until browned and fully cooked. Drain beef and return to pot. Add onion, continue cooking until soft. Add garlic and Italian seasoning, stir and cook until fragrant, about 30 seconds. Add broth, diced tomatoes, and cubed potatoes. Bring to a boil, reduce heat and simmer until potatoes are tender, about 15 minutes. Add mixed veggies, season with salt and pepper, cook for another 5 minutes until vegetables are warm. Serve hot.

Pro-Tip: You can use whatever variety of vegetables you prefer in this recipe, but most common is the green beans/corn/peas/carrots medley.

White Bean Chili *(6-8 servings)*

1 medium yellow onion, diced
1 tbsp. coconut oil
3 cloves garlic, minced
14.5 oz. container organic vegetable broth
4 oz. can diced green chiles, drained
½ tbsp. cumin
½ tsp. paprika
½ tsp. dried oregano

½ tsp. ground coriander
¼ tsp. cayenne
1 tbsp. sea salt
½ tsp. black pepper
12 oz. bag steam-in-a-bag cauliflower
8 oz. cream cheese
3 (15 oz.) cans cannellini beans, drained
12 oz. bag frozen corn, thawed

In a large pot, combine onion and coconut oil, cook on medium heat until onions are tender. Add garlic and continue cooking for another minute, add 2 cups of vegetable broth, chiles, all spices, and continue cooking for another 6-10 minutes. Cook cauliflower in microwave according to package directions. When cauliflower is done cooking, add to a blender along with remaining vegetable broth, cream cheese, and 1 can of cannellini beans. Puree soup until smooth, pour into pot. Add remaining two cans of beans and corn, cook for another 5 minutes. Serve warm.

Pro-Tip: switch out the regular cream cheese for dairy-free cream cheese as a healthier option.

Alfredo Sauce *(6-8 servings)*

1 cup butter
¼ cup gluten-free all-purpose flour (no XG)
2 cloves garlic, minced

4 cups half and half
½ cup grated parmesan
salt and pepper to taste

Melt butter in a large pot on medium heat. Whisk in flour and cook for another minute, add garlic and stir. Slowly whisk in half and half, continue cooking for about 10 minutes to allow sauce to thicken. When sauce has thickened, stir in salt and parmesan until cheese is melted and smooth.

BBQ Sauce *(16 servings)*

¾ cup brown sugar
¾ cup ketchup
¼ cup red wine vinegar
¼ cup water
½ tbsp. gluten-free Worcestershire

2 tbsp. Dijon mustard
1 tsp. paprika
1 tsp. salt
½ tsp. black pepper
1 dash hot pepper sauce (optional)

Combine all ingredients in a blender and puree until smooth. Store in airtight container in refrigerator for up to two weeks.

Bearnaise Sauce *(4-6 servings)*

¼ cup white wine vinegar
1 small shallot, peeled and minced
½ tsp. black pepper
4 tsp. chopped tarragon leaves

2 egg yolks
12 tbsp. butter
salt, to taste

Combine vinegar, shallot, pepper, and tarragon leaves in a small saucepan and cook over medium heat. Bring just to a boil, then reduce heat to a simmer for about 5 minutes, or until liquid has reduced by half. Remove from heat, set aside to cool. Melt butter in microwave until hot. In a blender, combine cooled mixture and egg yolks. Blend for about 5 seconds, just until combined. Turn on the blender to low/medium speed, then slowly stream the butter into mixture until it is emulsified, season with desired amount of salt. If the sauce is too thick, add some water to thin it out. Serve immediately over Chicken Cordon Bleu (p. 107), steak, seafood, or veggies.

I used to make Bearnaise Sauce with the little packets at the grocery store for convenience until I decided to look at the ingredients list. My disappointment screamed volumes as I stuck out my lower lip and put it back on the shelf. Thankfully, I learned from culinary school that making it at home wasn't impossible, I just had to make the effort. Let's get an A for effort.

Bechamel Sauce ♀ *(6-8 servings)*

1 cup butter   2 cups milk
½ cup gluten-free all-purpose flour (no XG)   salt and pepper to taste
2 cups chicken broth

Melt butter in a pot on medium heat. Whisk in flour and cook for another minute. Slowly whisk in chicken broth and milk, continue cooking for about 10 minutes to allow sauce to thicken. When sauce has thickened, add salt and pepper to taste.

Pro-Tip: this is a base cream sauce that goes with many, many recipes. You can basically slather this sauce on almost any dish and be happy as a pig in mud. For a dairy-free option, use plant-butter and about 1-1 ½ cups dairy-free milk.

Cauliflower Gravy ♀ *(4-6 servings)*

1 head cauliflower   2-4 tbsp. butter
½ cup chicken or vegetable broth   salt and pepper, to taste

Cut cauliflower into florets and boil or steam until tender. Place cauliflower in a blender, add chicken broth and butter. Puree until smooth, add more broth for a thinner consistency, season with salt and pepper. Serve warm.

Country Gravy ♀ *(6-8 servings)*

¼ cup butter   ½ tsp. salt
¼ cup gluten-free all-purpose flour (no XG)   ¼ tsp. garlic powder
1 tsp. black pepper   2 cups milk

Heat butter in a saucepan on medium heat. When butter has melted, whisk in flour and cook for about 1 minute. Add pepper, salt, and garlic powder, whisk again. Slowly add milk, whisking constantly to break up any clumps. Continue to cook until gravy has thickened, serve warm.

Enchilada Sauce ♀ *(6-8 servings)*

½ cup vegetable oil   3 cups water
¼ cup gluten-free all-purpose flour (no XG)   ½ tsp. ground cumin
½ cup chili powder   ½ tsp. garlic powder
15 oz. can tomato sauce   ½ tsp. onion powder

Heat oil in a saucepan over medium heat. Whisk in flour and chili powder, continue cooking for another minute. Add remaining ingredients, continue to stir while cooking another 10 minutes, or until sauce has thickened.

Garlic Sauce (12-16 servings)

½ cup garlic cloves, peeled
1 tsp. salt

1 ½ cups oil (canola or safflower)
¼ cup lemon juice

Slice garlic cloves in half, transfer to a food processor with salt and process until garlic becomes finely minced. Scrape down the sides of the food processor. While the food processor is running, slowly add 2 tablespoons of oil. Scrape down sides and repeat process until garlic starts to look creamy. Increase speed of pouring in oil and alternate with adding lemon juice until all of both are incorporated. This will take about 5 minutes to complete. Spoon sauce into a glass container, cover with paper towel and place in refrigerator overnight. The next day, replace paper towel with airtight lid, store in refrigerator for up to 3 months.

Pro-Tip: for a healthier option, use liquid coconut oil. Many brands of solid coconut oil have a stronger coconut smell and the sauce won't stay smooth, whereas the liquid coconut oil used in this recipe has a neutral smell and will stay smooth.

Hollandaise Sauce (4-6 servings)

½ cup butter
3 egg yolks
1 tbsp. lemon juice

1 tsp. Dijon mustard
¼ tsp. salt
1/8 tsp. cayenne

Melt butter in microwave until hot. In a blender, add egg yolks, lemon juice, mustard, salt, and cayenne. Blend for about 5 seconds, just until combined. Turn on the blender to low/medium speed, then slowly stream the butter into mixture until it's emulsified. Serve warm, goes well with steak, seafood, and vegetables.

Marsala Sauce (6-8 servings)

1 cup butter
1 cup gluten-free all-purpose flour (no XG)
3 cloves garlic, minced
2 cups marsala cooking wine
3 cups chicken broth
2 cups heavy cream

¼ cup olive oil
2 lbs. mushrooms
¾ tsp. salt
¼ tsp. black pepper
¾ cup grated parmesan

Melt butter in a pot on medium heat. Whisk in flour and cook for another minute, add garlic and stir. Slowly whisk in marsala, followed by chicken broth, then heavy cream. Continue cooking for about 10 minutes to allow sauce to thicken, stirring occasionally. In a separate pan, sauté mushrooms in ¼ cup olive oil until tender, drain and set aside. When sauce has thickened, stir in salt, pepper, and parmesan until cheese is melted and smooth. Remove from heat, stir in mushrooms and serve warm over gluten-free pasta.

Meaty Marinara ♀ (6-8 servings)

1 lb. ground beef
28 oz. can crushed tomatoes
16 oz. can tomato sauce
6 oz. can tomato paste
2 tbsp. onion powder
3 cloves garlic, minced

2 tsp. dried oregano
2 tsp. dried basil
1 tsp. salt
½ tsp. black pepper
1 tbsp. sugar

Cook beef in a stock pot on medium heat. When beef is fully cooked and browned, drain and return to pot before adding all remaining ingredients. Cover and cook on low/medium heat and stir occasionally for about 20-30 minutes. Serve warm, store leftovers in refrigerator for up to 7 days or freezer for 6 months.

Shortcut: use 2 jars of storebought spaghetti sauce with meat!

Mornay Sauce ♀♀ (6-8 servings)

¼ cup butter
1/3 cup gluten-free all-purpose flour (no XG)
3 cups whole milk, divided
1 tsp. ground cloves

½ tsp. onion powder
1 bay leaf
2 oz. grated gruyere cheese
2 oz. grated parmesan cheese

Melt butter in a medium saucepan over low/medium heat. When butter has melted, whisk in the flour and cook for 1-2 minutes, whisking frequently. Slowly whisk in 2 ½ cups of the milk, whisking constantly to break up any lumps. Add the ground cloves and onion powder, whisk again. Add bay leaf and continue to cook for another 10 minutes, until sauce has thickened. Remove bay leaf, then add cheeses and stir until melted and smooth. Remove from heat, adjust consistency of sauce by adding remaining amount of milk. Serve warm.

Mushroom Gravy ♀♀ (6-8 servings)

¼ cup butter
16 oz. package sliced mushrooms
¼ cup gluten-free all-purpose flour (no XG)
4 cups beef stock

1/8 tsp. black pepper
¼ tsp. dried thyme
salt to taste

Melt butter in a medium saucepan on medium heat. Add mushrooms, stir occasionally and cook until tender, about 15 minutes. Add flour and stir, cook for another 5 minutes. Pour in 1 cup beef stock, stir briskly until incorporated. Pour in remaining stock, add pepper, thyme, and salt, stir again. Reduce heat to medium/low and cook for about 30 minutes until sauce has thickened, stirring often. Serve warm.

Pan Gravy 🍴 *(6-8 servings)*

Drippings from roasted meat*
¼ cup gluten-free all-purpose flour (no XG)

2 cups stock*
salt and pepper to taste

After roasting the meat, transfer it to a warmed platter and set aside. Skim the excess fat from the liquid in the roasting pan, scrape the bottom with a wooden spoon to get the caramelized pan juices, then pour liquid into a medium saucepan over medium heat. Add flour and whisk together well, cook for about 1-2 minutes. Slowly add stock to the saucepan and whisk very well to break up any clumps and bring to a boil. Whisk constantly while sauce is cooking until gravy reduces and has thickened. Pour gravy through a fine mesh strainer before serving, if desire.

🍴 **Pro-Tip:** The type of meat will set the stage for this recipe: roast beef, chicken, turkey, pork loin, or other cut of non-brined meat. If you're using beef, use beef stock to make the gravy, chicken broth with roasted chicken or turkey, etc. Add the stock slowly and adjust amount as necessary to reach desired consistency. More liquid for a thinner gravy, less for a thicker gravy.

Pesto Sauce 🍴 *(4-6 servings)*

2 cups basil leaves, stems removed
2 tbsp. pine nuts
2 cloves garlic, minced

½ cup extra virgin olive oil
½ cup parmesan cheese

Combine basil leaves, pine nuts, and garlic in a food processor and process until finely minced. Slowly drizzle in olive oil and continue to process until smooth. Add parmesan and process just until combined. Store in refrigerator for up to 7 days or freezer for up to 4 months.

Red Pepper Butter 🍴 *(12-16 servings)*

1 lb. butter, softened

¼ cup roasted red bell pepper, minced

Combine butter and diced bell pepper in a small mixing bowl, beat with electric mixer until smooth. Spoon on top of a piece of plastic wrap, cover completely and roll into a log. Store in refrigerator to set before using in recipes. When ready to use, slice desired amount from log. Use this to sauté veggies, in baked potatoes, spread on bread, or top on steaks.

🍴 **Pro-Tip:** grab a jar of roasted red bell peppers for a quick and easy version of this recipe!

Remoulade Sauce ⚲ *(10-12 servings)*

1 ¼ cups mayonnaise
2 tbsp. spicy brown mustard
1 tbsp. paprika
1 tsp. Creole or Cajun seasoning

2 tsp. prepared horseradish
1 tsp. pickle juice
1 tsp. hot sauce
1 clove garlic, minced

Combine all ingredients in a small mixing bowl and stir together well. Let chill in refrigerator for at least two hours before serving so the flavors have a chance to come together. Store in refrigerator for up to two weeks.

Spaghetti Sauce ⚲ *(6-8 servings)*

28 oz. can crushed tomatoes
16 oz. can tomato sauce
6 oz. can tomato paste
2 tbsp. onion powder
3 cloves garlic, minced

2 tsp. dried oregano
2 tsp. dried basil
1 tsp. salt
½ tsp. black pepper
1 tbsp. sugar

Combine all ingredients in a pot and cook on low/medium heat for about 10-15 minutes until hot. Serve immediately, or transfer to glass airtight containers and store in refrigerator for up to 1 week or freezer for 6 months.

Strawberry Sauce ⚲ *(8-10 servings)*

3 cups frozen strawberries, thawed

1 tbsp. granulated sugar

Throw strawberries in a medium saucepan on medium heat. When strawberries start to heat up, mash well with a potato masher or fork. Add sugar and stir, continue cooking for about 5 minutes. Remove from heat and set aside to cool. Store in refrigerator for up to 1 week or in freezer for 6 months.

Tartar Sauce ⚲ *(6-8 servings)*

1 cup mayonnaise
¾ cup dill pickles, finely chopped
1 tbsp. freshly parsley, finely chopped

1 tsp. lemon juice
1 tsp. granulated sugar
¼ tsp. black pepper

Combine all ingredients in a small mixing bowl and stir together until well-combined. Store in refrigerator for up to 1 week.

Veggie Marinara *(4-6 servings)*

2 tbsp. olive oil
2 medium zucchini
8 oz. package cleaned, sliced mushrooms
28 oz. can crushed tomatoes

3 cloves garlic, minced
2 tbsp. onion powder
2 tbsp. Italian seasoning
Salt and pepper to taste

In a pot on medium heat, add olive oil. Cut zucchini into ½ inch pieces, add to pot and cook until tender, about 5-10 minutes. Add mushrooms and continue cooking until vegetables are soft. Add garlic and cook for 1 minute, then add crushed tomatoes, onion powder, and Italian seasoning. Reduce heat to low medium, cover and cook for another 10 minutes, stirring occasionally. Serve warm over pasta, Pan Fried Eggplant (p. 192), or use in Vegetarian Lasagna (p. 204).

Apple Pecan Salad *(4 servings)*

1 (10 oz.) bag mixed greens salad
1 apple, cored and chopped
½ cup chopped pecans

¼ cup mayonnaise
1 tbsp. Dijon mustard
1 tbsp. honey

Preheat oven to 350 degrees. Spread pecans on a small baking sheet, place in oven. Roast for 3-4 minutes, just until you smell that delicious roasted flavor. Remove from oven, set aside to cool. In a large bowl, combine salad, chopped apples and pecans. In a small separate bowl, whisk together mayonnaise, mustard, and honey. Pour over salad, toss well to coat. Add your choice of cooked chicken, shrimp, or deli meat if desired.

Asian Chicken Salad *(2 servings)*

2 cups cooked brown rice, cooled
1 cup cooked chicken, shredded
2 cups chopped baby Bok choy
1 cup fresh spinach leaves
½ cup grated carrots

½ cup diced celery
¼ cup diced red bell pepper
¼ cup sliced green onions
¼ cup cilantro, chopped
Asian Dressing (p. 97)

Combine all ingredients in a large mixing bowl, mix thoroughly. Serve immediately.

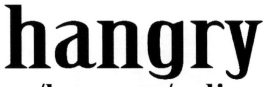

hangry
/han-gree/ adj.
A state of anger resulting
from a lack of food.

Big Mac Salad ⅄ *(4-6 servings)*

1 lb. ground beef
1 tbsp. Montreal steak seasoning
8 oz. romaine lettuce
1 cup diced tomatoes

½ cup diced pickles
1 cup grated cheddar cheese
Thousand Island Dressing (p. 99)

Cook ground beef in a skillet on medium heat, stirring occasionally and cook until browned. Drain and return to pan, add seasoning and stir, set aside. Chop romaine lettuce and arrange in one large bowl or single bowls. Spoon ground beef on top, along with diced tomatoes, diced pickles, cheddar cheese, and dressing. Serve immediately.

Broccoli Salad ⅄ *(4-6 servings)*

1 (12 oz.) bag fresh broccoli florets
¼ cup real bacon bits
½ cup grated sharp cheddar cheese

½ cup mayonnaise
1 tbsp. sugar
1 tbsp. vinegar

In a medium size mixing bowl, whisk together mayonnaise, sugar, and vinegar until smooth. Make sure the broccoli florets are cut into bite size pieces. Add broccoli, bacon bits, and cheese to mixing bowl. Stir to combine well, store in refrigerator. Serve cold.

Caesar Salad ⅄ *(2-4 servings)*

8 oz. romaine lettuce
1/3 cup grated parmesan

Caesar Dressing (p. 97)
Garlic Croutons (p. 99)

Rinse, dry, and chop or tear lettuce into bite size pieces and place in a large serving bowl. Sprinkle parmesan cheese and croutons on top, then add dressing and toss together well. Serve immediately.

Candied Pecan Salad ⅄ *(2-4 servings)*

8 oz. mixed greens
1 pear, cored and chopped
1 cup Candied Pecans

2/3 cup dried cranberries
4 oz. feta cheese crumbles
Vinaigrette Dressing (p. 99)

Place greens in a large serving bowl or divide among individual plates. Sprinkle chopped pears, candied pecans, dried cranberries, and feta cheese on top. Drizzle with dressing and serve immediately.

For Candied Pecans: preheat oven to 250 degrees. In a small mixing bowl, whisk 1 egg white with 1 tbsp. water. Add ¼ cup sugar, 1 tsp. cinnamon, ¼ tsp. salt and whisk again. Add 1 lb. pecan halves and stir. Spread on baking sheet and bake for about 60 minutes, stirring occasionally until evenly browned.

Caprese Salad *(4-6 servings)*

3 medium size tomatoes, sliced
2 (8 oz.) packages fresh mozzarella, sliced
1 tbsp. olive oil

1 tsp. dried basil
Salt and pepper
Balsamic Vinegar

Alternately lay slices of tomatoes on a plate with slices of mozzarella, overlapping each other. In a small dish, stir together the olive oil and dried basil. Drizzle oil over tomatoes and mozzarella. Lightly sprinkle with salt and pepper. Drizzle with balsamic vinegar.

Cobb Salad *(4-6 servings)*

1 large head iceberg lettuce
3 hard-boiled eggs, chopped
½ cup real bacon bits
3 cups cooked chicken, diced

2 tomatoes, seeded and chopped
1 avocado, peeled, pitted and diced
1 cup grated cheddar cheese
Ranch Dressing (p. 98)

Rinse, dry, and chop lettuce into bite-size pieces before placing in one large serving bowl or individual bowls. Sprinkle eggs, bacon, chicken, tomatoes, avocado, and cheddar cheese on top of lettuce. Serve with Ranch dressing and enjoy immediately.

Cucumber Salad *(4 servings)*

1 lb. seedless cucumbers, thinly sliced
½ tbsp. granulated sugar
½ tbsp. sea salt

2 ½ tbsp. red wine vinegar
½ small onion, thinly sliced

In a medium size bowl, combine cucumbers, sugar, and salt. Toss together well and let sit for 5 minutes. Add vinegar and onion, stir together and refrigerate for at least 10 minutes before serving.

Egg Salad *(4-6 servings)*

1 dozen eggs
½ cup mayonnaise
2 tsp. Dijon mustard

¾ tsp. salt, divided
¼ tsp. pepper

Put eggs and ½ teaspoon salt in a large pot with enough water to cover all the eggs. Heat the pot on high heat on the stove, bring to a rolling boil (lots and lots of bubbles). Leave the pot on the burner but turn off the heat and place a cover on the pot. Let sit for 15-17 minutes. Take the pot off stove and run cold water into pot to cool eggs. Gently tap each egg on side of pot to create a crack, then peel shells off eggs and rinse thoroughly. Place eggs on a cutting board, chop into small pieces and transfer to a medium size mixing bowl. Add mayonnaise, mustard, salt, and pepper. Stir well to combine, store in refrigerator.

Greek Salad 🍴 *(4-6 servings)*

1 English cucumber, seeded
1 yellow bell pepper, seeded
2 cups halved cherry tomatoes

1/3 cup thinly sliced red onions
1/3 cup pitted Kalamata olives
5 oz. feta cheese, cut into ½ inch cubes

Slice cucumber into ¼ inch pieces and bell pepper into ½ inch pieces. In a medium size bowl, combine all ingredients and toss together. Add Greek Vinaigrette and toss together again, set aside for 30 minutes before serving at room temperature.

For the Greek Vinaigrette 🍴

¼ cup extra-virgin olive oil
3 tbsp. red wine vinegar
1 garlic clove, minced
½ tsp. dried oregano

½ tsp. Dijon mustard
¼ tsp. sea salt
¼ tsp. black pepper

Combine all ingredients in a small bowl and whisk together well before pouring over Greek salad.

Macaroni Salad 🍴 *(6-8 servings)*

16 oz. gluten-free elbow macaroni noodles
1 cup mayonnaise
½ cup granulated sugar
2 tbsp. distilled white vinegar

2 tbsp. Dijon mustard
¼ cup diced onion
¼ cup diced green bell peppers
¼ cup real bacon bits

Cook macaroni noodles according to package directions to al dente. While noodles are cooking, combine the mayonnaise, sugar, vinegar, and mustard in a medium size mixing bowl. Whisk together well. When noodles are done cooking, drain and run cold water over them until they are cool. Add noodles, onion, bell peppers, and bacon bits to bowl. Stir together, cover and place in refrigerator to set for at least 4 hours before serving.

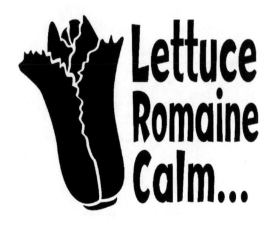

Potato Salad ♛ *(6-8 servings)*

2 ½ lbs. Yukon Gold potatoes
1 cup mayonnaise
½ cup sweet pickle relish
1 tbsp. Dijon mustard
½ tbsp. apple cider vinegar
½ tbsp. celery seeds

¼ tsp. paprika
2 hard-boiled eggs, peeled and chopped
2 celery stalks, diced
¼ cup sweet onion, diced
½ tbsp. chopped fresh dill
salt and pepper to taste

Cut the potatoes into quarters and place in a large stockpot before filling with cold water. You'll want the water to come up to about 1 inch higher than the potatoes. Set the pot on high heat and bring to a boil. Once the water starts to boil, add 1 tablespoon salt and cook for about 15 minutes, until potatoes are fork tender. While the potatoes are cooking, combine mayonnaise, relish, mustard, apple cider vinegar, celery seeds, paprika, salt, and pepper in a medium size mixing bowl. Stir together well. When the potatoes are done cooking, drain all the water and chop into ½ inch chunks. Place potatoes in a large bowl, pour dressing on top of potatoes and gently stir together until potatoes are coated. Add the eggs, celery, onion, and dill, stir together again. Season with desired amount of salt and pepper, taste to make any adjustments. Cover and refrigerate for at least 4 hours to let flavors marinate. Store in refrigerator for one week.

Quinoa Kale Salad ♛ *(4-6 servings)*

2 bunches organic kale
juice from 1 lemon
2 tbsp. olive oil
½ tsp. sea salt
2 cups cooked quinoa, cooled

¾ cup chopped walnuts
¾ cup raw pumpkin seeds
½ cup diced sun-dried tomatoes
1 batch Lemon Tahini Dressing (p. 98)

In a large mixing bowl, combine kale, lemon juice, olive oil, and sea salt. Massage kale with clean hands for 5-7 minutes, until it becomes dark green and soft. Add cooked quinoa, walnuts, sun-dried tomatoes, and dressing. Toss together until well-combined, store in refrigerator for up to 5 days.

The massage step for this recipe is crucial! You know how you feel like a puddle of goo after a good massage? That's what you're looking for with massaging the kale. Since kale is naturally rough in texture, massaging it into a puddle of goo will make it tender and soft, ready to be eaten.

Salad Niçoise ♙ *(4-6 servings)*

1 red onion, thinly sliced
1 lb. small red potatoes
Salt and pepper to taste
8 oz. green beans
2 heads Boston or butter lettuce

2 (5 oz.) cans tuna, drained
3 small ripe tomatoes
6 hard-boiled eggs, sliced
¼ cup Niçoise olives
2 tbsp. capers

Place onion slices in a small bowl and drizzle with 3 tablespoons vinaigrette, set aside. Place potatoes in a large pot and cover with 2 inches of water, then add 1 tablespoon salt. Heat on high and bring to a boil, then lower heat to maintain a simmer for 10-12 minutes, until potatoes are fork tender. While potatoes are cooking, fill a medium size pot halfway with water, add 2 teaspoons of salt and bring to a boil on high heat. Add green beans to boiling water and cook for about 3-5 minutes. Drain and rinse with cold water. When potatoes are done cooking, drain and cut into halves or quarters, place in a bowl and drizzle with ¼ cup vinaigrette. Chop or tear lettuce into bite-size pieces and arrange a bed on a large serving platter. Mound tuna in center of platter, sprinkle tomatoes and onions around tuna. Arrange potatoes and green beans on the edge of lettuce, followed by the hard boiled eggs, and olives. Drizzle with remaining vinaigrette, sprinkle with capers and serve immediately.

For the Vinaigrette ♙

1/3 cup lemon juice
¾ cup extra-virgin olive oil
3 tbsp. minced shallot
2 tbsp. chopped fresh basil

1 tbsp. chopped fresh thyme
2 tsp. chopped fresh oregano
1 tsp. Dijon mustard
salt and pepper to taste

Combine all ingredients in a small bowl and whisk together well before using in recipe.

Seven Layer Salad ♙ *(6-8 servings)*

2 (10 oz.) bags salad greens
4.5 oz. package real bacon bits
½ cup diced onion
10 oz. bag frozen peas, thawed

2 cups grated cheddar cheese
2 cups mayonnaise
½ cup milk
1 oz. packet ranch dressing mix

Dump both bags of salad into a large bowl or trifle dish. Sprinkle bacon bits, diced onions and peas on top. In a small mixing bowl, whisk the mayonnaise, milk, and ranch dressing; spoon over salad into even layer. Sprinkle grated cheese on top, cover with plastic wrap and set in refrigerator for at least 2 hours before serving.

Taco Salad (4-6 servings)

1 lb. ground beef
1.25 oz. packet taco seasoning
¼ cup water
1 (10 oz.) bag salad greens

Grated cheddar cheese
Catalina Dressing (p. 98)
1 bag corn chips (like Fritos®)

Cook the hamburger in a skillet on medium heat, mashing down to break up meat, cooking until completely browned. Drain meat and return to pot, add water and taco seasoning, stir well to combine. Lay salad in a large bowl or individual bowls, top with cheese, dressing, corn chips and beef. Feel free to add other veggies, like chopped tomatoes and onions, cooked beans, salsa, corn, guacamole, etc.

Asian Dressing (4-6 servings)

¼ cup sunflower seed butter
¼ cup avocado oil
2 tbsp. lime juice
2 tbsp. rice vinegar
2 tbsp. tamari (or coconut aminos)

1 tsp. sesame oil
2 tbsp. grated ginger
2 cloves garlic, minced
1 tbsp. honey
1 tsp. red chili flakes

Combine all ingredients in a blender and puree until smooth. Add water if needed for a thinner consistency. Store in refrigerator for up to 5 days.

Avocado Ranch Dressing (10-12 servings)

1 avocado
1 cup milk

1 cup mayonnaise
1 oz. powdered ranch packet

Slice avocado and remove pit. Scoop out pulp, combine in a blender with milk and puree until smooth. In a medium size mixing bowl, combine avocado mixture with mayonnaise and ranch packet, whisk together well. Add more milk for a thinner consistency, if desired. Store in refrigerator for up to one week.

Caesar Dressing (4-6 servings)

½ cup mayonnaise
1 garlic clove, minced
2 tsp. lemon juice
1 tsp. Dijon mustard
½ tsp. Worcestershire sauce

1/8 teaspoon salt
1/3 cup finely grated parmesan
1 tbsp. water
1/8 teaspoon black pepper

Combine all ingredients in a mixing bowl and whisk together very well. Store in refrigerator for up to one week.

Catalina Dressing *(4-6 servings)*

1/3 cup red wine vinegar
½ cup ketchup
½ cup honey
½ cup olive oil

2 tsp. coconut aminos
1 tsp. paprika
½ tsp. onion powder
½ tsp. garlic powder

Combine all ingredients in a small mixing bowl and whisk together well. Store in refrigerator for up to one week.

Honey Mustard Dressing *(6-8 servings)*

1 cup mayonnaise
½ cup honey

½ cup Dijon mustard

Combine all ingredients in a small mixing bowl and whisk together well. Store in refrigerator for up to one week.

Lemon Tahini Dressing *(4-6 servings)*

½ cup water
½ cup olive oil
½ cup tahini
juice from 1 lemon

2 tbsp. coconut aminos
2 cloves garlic, minced
½ tsp. sea salt

Combine all ingredients in a small blender or bullet, blend until smooth. Store in refrigerator for up to one week.

Ranch Dressing *(6-8 servings)*

½ cup mayonnaise
½ cup sour cream
½ cup buttermilk
1 tsp. dried dillweed
½ tsp. dried parsley
½ tsp. dried chives

¼ tsp. onion powder
½ tsp. garlic powder
¼ tsp. salt
1/8 tsp. black pepper
1-3 tsp. lemon juice

Combine all ingredients in a mixing bowl and whisk together very well. Adjust amount of lemon juice to taste. Store in refrigerator for up to one week.

Raspberry Vinaigrette ⸙ *(8-10 servings)*

1 ½ cups raspberries
½ cup olive oil
¼ cup red wine vinegar

1 small shallot, diced
1 tsp. Dijon mustard
¼ tsp. salt

Combine all ingredients in a blender or food processor and puree until smooth. Pour through a fine mesh strainer to catch seeds. Store in refrigerator for up to one week.

Thousand Island Dressing ⸙ *(4-6 servings)*

½ cup mayonnaise
2 tbsp. ketchup
1 tbsp. white vinegar
2 tsp. granulated sugar

2 tsp. sweet pickle relish
½ tsp. onion powder
1/8 tsp. salt
pinch of black pepper

Combine all ingredients in a small mixing bowl and whisk together well. Store in refrigerator for up to one week.

Vinaigrette ⸙ *(4-6 servings)*

¼ cup balsamic vinegar
¼ cup olive oil

¼ cup Dijon mustard
¼ cup honey

Combine all ingredients in a small mixing bowl and whisk together well. Store in refrigerator for up to one week.

Garlic Croutons ⸙ *(10-12 servings)*

1 loaf stale gluten-free bread
¼ cup melted butter or olive oil
1 tsp. Italian seasoning

½ tsp. garlic powder
½ tsp. salt

Preheat oven to 375 degrees. Cut bread into ¼ inch chunks, place in a large mixing bowl. Add melted butter or olive oil, Italian seasoning, garlic powder and salt, toss together to combine well. Spread into a large baking pan and bake in oven for 10-12 minutes, or until golden brown. When done baking, remove from oven and let cool slightly before transferring to airtight container. Store for up to two weeks.

Poultry

BBQ Chicken Pizza *(3-4 servings)*

1 gluten-free pizza crust*
1 tbsp. olive oil

¾ cup BBQ Pulled Chicken (below)
2 cups Monterey Jack cheese

Preheat oven to 350 degrees (or whatever temperature your pizza dough instructions tell you). Place prepared pizza crust on cookie sheet or pizza pan. Brush pizza crust with olive oil. Spread BBQ Pulled Chicken on crust into an even layer. Sprinkle grated cheese on top, bake pizza in oven for 15-20 minutes, or until cheese is melted. Remove from oven, slice into pieces, and serve warm.

Pro-Tip: for your pizza crust, you have several options. You can buy the pre-made gluten-free pizza crusts found with traditional pizza crusts, in the frozen section, or make your own Pizza Dough on page 223!

BBQ Pulled Chicken *(6-8 servings)*

2 lbs. boneless chicken thighs
12 oz. bottle gluten-free BBQ sauce

1 cup Ranch dressing
½ cup light brown sugar

Spray 4-quart slow cooker with cooking spray, then place chicken inside. In a small mixing bowl, whisk together BBQ sauce, ranch dressing and sugar. Pour on top of chicken; cook on low for 4 hours. Using two forks, shred chicken. Serve warm.

Breaded Baked Chicken *(4 servings)*

4 (5 oz.) boneless chicken breasts
1/3 cup mayonnaise

1 cup gluten-free seasoned breadcrumbs

Preheat oven to 375 degrees. Pour breadcrumbs in a bowl and set aside. Place one piece of chicken on a plate and generously brush mayonnaise on one side. Place chicken, mayonnaise side down into breadcrumbs. Press gently. Brush more mayonnaise on the top of chicken, flip over in breadcrumbs and press again, making sure breadcrumbs cover both sides of chicken. Repeat process with each piece of chicken, placing each one in 9x13 inch baking dish. Bake in oven for 25-30 minutes, or until chicken is cooked (until juices run clear, NO PINK when chicken is cut, and/or thickest part of chicken reaches 165 degrees). Serve warm.

Pro-Tip: for crunchier chicken, pound chicken breasts using a meat mallet in between two pieces of plastic wrap to ½ inch thickness. This will decrease your cooking time and the breading will give more crunch since the meat is thinner.

Buffalo Stuffed Sweet Potatoes *(4-6 servings)*

4 sweet potatoes
¾ cup gluten-free hot sauce
2 tbsp. butter
1 tsp. sea salt
1 tsp. garlic powder
½ tsp. cayenne
1 tbsp. cornstarch
2 cups cooked, shredded chicken
chopped green onions

Preheat oven to 400 degrees. Using a fork, prick the sweet potatoes all over before placing on a foil-lined baking sheet. Bake until the sweet potatoes are tender, about 45-60 minutes (depends on the size of sweet potatoes). While the sweet potatoes are baking, combine hot sauce, butter, salt, garlic powder, and cayenne in a small saucepan over medium heat and whisk together. Combine cornstarch with 1 tablespoon water and whisk very well before pouring into sauce. Add chicken and continue cooking until sauce has thickened and chicken is hot. When sweet potatoes are nice and tender, top with chicken mixture and garnish with chopped green onions. Serve hot.

Cajun Chicken *(4 servings)*

4 (5 oz.) boneless chicken breasts
2 tbsp. Cajun seasoning
¼ cup butter
2 cloves garlic, minced
½ cup chicken broth
½ cup heavy cream
¼ cup grated parmesan
chopped parsley for garnish

Season both sides of each chicken breast with Cajun seasoning. Heat butter on medium heat in a large skillet pan and sear chicken for 4-6 minutes on each side, until golden or internal temperature reaches 165 degrees. Remove chicken from pan and set aside on a plate. Add garlic cloves to pan, cook for 1 minute until fragrant. Add chicken broth and heavy cream, scrape brown bits from bottom of pan. Reduce heat to low, simmer for 2-3 minutes and stir occasionally. Add grated parmesan and stir, then place chicken breasts back in pan with sauce until heated through. Serve hot.

Carolina Reuben *(2 servings)*

4 pieces gluten-free sandwich bread
2 tbsp. Thousand Island Dressing (p. 99)
6-8 slices deli turkey
2 slices Swiss cheese
½ cup prepared coleslaw
1 tbsp. butter, softened

Set oven to (high) broil. Place all four pieces of bread on baking sheet. Spread 1 tablespoon Thousand Island dressing on two pieces of bread. Place 3-4 slices turkey on bread topped with dressing, followed by 1 piece of cheese on each. On remaining pieces of bread, spread ½ tablespoon of butter. Place pan in oven and broil for 1-2 minutes, until cheese is melted and buttered bread is lightly toasted. Remove pan from oven. Spoon ¼ cup coleslaw over melted Swiss, place remaining bread slices (butter side up) on top. Serve immediately.

Cheesy Chicken Enchiladas ⬩ *(8 servings)*

8 oz. sour cream
1 tbsp. taco seasoning
1 lb. grated Mexican blend cheese, divided

1 lb. cooked chicken, diced
16 corn tortillas

Preheat oven to 350 degrees. In a medium sized mixing bowl, whisk together sour cream and taco seasoning until mixed well. Set aside 1 cup grated cheese for topping. Add chicken and remaining cheese, stir until well combined. Scoop 1/3 cup of chicken mixture into tortilla. Spread into an even layer in the shape of a rectangle, about 1 inch from the sides of the tortilla. Tuck in the sides and roll up tortilla, place seam side down in greased 9x13 inch baking dish. Repeat process with remaining tortillas. Pour Enchilada Sauce (p. 86) on top and sprinkle with 1 cup cheese. Bake in oven for 30 minutes, serve hot.

Chicken Alfredo ⬩ *(6-8 servings)*

1 cup unsalted butter
¼ cup gluten-free all-purpose flour (no XG)
1 tbsp. minced garlic
1 quart half and half
4 oz. grated parmesan*

1 tsp. sea salt
1 lb. gluten-free penne pasta
1 lb. cooked chicken, diced
1 cup grated mozzarella cheese

Melt butter in a pot on medium heat. Whisk in flour and cook for another minute, add garlic and stir. Slowly whisk in half and half, continue cooking for about 10 minutes to allow sauce to thicken. Meanwhile, cook pasta according to package directions for al dente and drain. When sauce has thickened, stir in salt and parmesan until cheese is melted and smooth. Remove from heat, stir in chicken and cooked pasta. Spoon into serving bowls or plate and top with grated mozzarella cheese, if desired.

⬩ **Pro-Tip:** grab a wedge of parmesan and grate it yourself. The texture and quality are significantly better, especially in sauces, since it doesn't have the added preservatives.

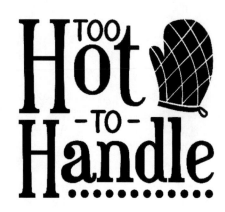

Chicken and Broccoli Tortellini ⅓ (8-10 servings)

1 lb. butter
¾ cup gluten-free all-purpose flour
½ gallon half and half
1 ½ tbsp. garlic powder
1 tbsp. sea salt

4 oz. grated parmesan
24 oz. frozen gluten-free cheese tortellini
1 ½ lbs. cooked chicken, diced
1 lb. broccoli florets
2 cups grated mozzarella cheese

Preheat oven to 350 degrees. Melt butter in a pot on medium heat. Whisk in flour and cook for another minute, add garlic and stir. Slowly whisk in half and half, continue cooking for about 10 minutes to allow sauce to thicken. Meanwhile, cook tortellini according to package directions for al dente and drain. Cook broccoli florets in boiling water for 3 minutes, drain. When sauce has thickened, stir in salt and parmesan until cheese is melted and smooth. Remove from heat, stir in chicken and cooked pasta. Spoon into greased 9x13 inch baking dish, top with mozzarella. Bake for 25-30 minutes, or until hot. Serve immediately.

Pro-Tip: this recipe can be made to serve immediately without baking, or with slapping on all that extra mozzarella on top to bake. The choice is yours.

Chicken and Dumplings ⅓ (6-8 servings)

1 cooked rotisserie chicken
4 cups chicken broth
1 lb. frozen mixed vegetables
2 bay leaves
1 tbsp. dried thyme
1 tbsp. onion powder
½ tsp. sea salt

2 cups milk
6 tbsp. cornstarch
1 ½ cups gluten-free Bisquick®
2 eggs, beaten
2/3 cup milk
¼ cup butter, melted

Pull meat from rotisserie chicken and throw in a pot with chicken broth, mixed vegetables, bay leaves, thyme, onion powder, and sea salt. Bring to a boil over medium heat. In a small bowl, combine milk and cornstarch, whisk together well until cornstarch is dissolved. Pour mixture into pot and stir until well combined. Continue to boil, stirring occasionally. In a medium size mixing bowl, combine Bisquick®, beaten eggs, milk, and melted butter. Stir until combined, batter will be sticky. Using a small ice cream scoop, drop scoops of batter into chicken broth mixture. Reduce heat to low and cook for 10 minutes, then cover and cook for an additional 15 minutes. Remove pot from heat and serve warm.

Chicken and Rice ♙♙ *(6-8 servings)*

2 lb. bone-in chicken breasts
5 cups water
2 tbsp. butter

1 tsp. salt
2 cups long-grain white rice
½ tsp. pepper

Combine chicken breasts, water, butter, and salt in an Instant Pot®. Secure lid and pressure cook on high for 10 minutes. When finished, allow pressure to release naturally for 5 minutes. Transfer chicken to cutting board, discard bones and break chicken into pieces, place in a bowl. Add rice to pot with liquid, secure lid and cook on high pressure for 3 minutes, then natural release for 10 minutes. Open lid, add chicken, pepper, and more salt if needed. Stir together and serve warm.

Chicken Bacon Ranch Casserole ♙ *(6-8 servings)*

2 lbs. broccoli florets
2 lbs. cooked chicken, diced
½ cup real bacon bits
8 oz. sour cream

1 cup mayonnaise
1 cup milk
3 tbsp. powdered ranch dressing
1 lb. grated cheddar cheese

Preheat oven to 350 degrees. Cook broccoli florets in boiling water for 3 minutes, drain. Spread broccoli into a greased 9x13 inch baking dish, sprinkle with diced chicken and bacon. In a medium size mixing bowl, combine sour cream, mayonnaise, milk, and powdered ranch dressing. Whisk together well, then pour on top of chicken mixture in dish. Sprinkle with cheddar and bake for 30-35 minutes. Serve warm.

Chicken Bog ♙♙♙ *(10-12 servings)*

4-5 lb. whole chicken
2 ribs celery, diced
1 yellow onion, diced
3 cloves garlic, minced

¼ cup butter
4 cups long grain rice
14 oz. package cooked sausage, sliced
salt and pepper, to taste

Remove and discard chicken innards, then place the chicken in a large stockpot. Add celery, onion, and garlic to pot. Fill pot with just enough water to cover the chicken, add 2 teaspoons salt and ½ teaspoon black pepper and stir. Simmer the chicken for about 45-60 minutes, or until cooked through and chicken reaches internal temperature of 165 degrees F. Do not boil chicken, it will cause it to be dry. When chicken is done cooking, remove to a large plate or serving platter to cool. Remove and shred the meat, discard bones, skin, and neck. Set meat aside. Pour the broth through a fine mesh strainer and set aside, you'll need the broth for later. In a medium stockpot, melt butter on medium heat. When melted, add sliced sausage and cook just until browned. Add 8 cups of reserved broth and bring to a rolling boil. Add rice and chicken, stir well. Reduce heat to a simmer, cover and continue cooking for about 20 minutes until rice is tender. Season with more salt and pepper as desired and add more broth if needed. Serve immediately.

Chicken Broccoli Casserole 🍴 (6-8 servings)

2 ½ cups chicken broth
1 tbsp. butter
1 ¼ cups long grain white rice, uncooked
1 lb. frozen broccoli florets, thawed
10.5 oz. can gluten-free cream of chicken soup
2 cups cooked chicken, diced

½ cup milk
½ cup sour cream
2 cups grated cheddar cheese, divided
1 cup gluten-free breadcrumbs
2 tbsp. butter, melted

Preheat oven to 350 degrees. Combine chicken broth, butter, and rice in a pot and bring to a boil, then reduce to simmer. Cover and cook for about 15 minutes, until rice is puffed. Transfer cooked rice to a large mixing bowl, add broccoli florets, cream of chicken soup, chicken, milk, sour cream, and 1 cup cheese. Stir together well, then spoon into a greased 9x13 inch baking dish. Sprinkle remaining cheese on top. Combine gluten-free breadcrumbs and melted butter together, toss together and sprinkle on top of cheese. Bake in oven for 30-35 minutes, let sit for five minutes before serving.

Chicken Cordon Bleu 🍴🍴🍴 (4 servings)

4 large boneless, skinless chicken breasts
4 slices Swiss cheese
4 slices ham
1 cup gluten-free all-purpose flour (no XG)
1 teaspoon paprika

1 tsp. salt
½ tsp. black pepper
2 eggs, lightly beaten
1 cup gluten-free breadcrumbs
½ cup grated parmesan

Preheat oven to 350 degrees. First, trim your chicken breast of excess fat. Place 1 piece of plastic wrap both under and over the chicken, then pound it to 1/4 inch thick using the flat side of a meat mallet. Place 1 piece of ham and 1 piece of Swiss cheese on top, making sure it's not the same width as the chicken. Roll the chicken up tightly with the ham and Swiss, making sure to tuck in the sides. Repeat process with other pieces of chicken, place in a greased 9x13 inch baking dish and in refrigerator for about 15 minutes. Prepare your dredging station: Three containers for seasoned flour, egg wash, and breadcrumbs/parmesan. Combine the flour, paprika, salt and pepper in a shallow bowl. Combine eggs with 2 tbsp. water in another shallow bowl and whisk together. In third shallow bowl, combine breadcrumbs and parmesan, stir together well.

First, roll chicken in seasoned flour, then egg wash, and finally in the breadcrumbs/parmesan mixture. Make sure the entire piece of chicken is covered by all three. Return to refrigerator for another 15 minutes. In a sauté pan, fill with canola oil, about 1 inch deep. Turn heat to low/medium. Make sure oil is hot before placing chickens in there to fry. Fry to a golden brown on each side just until lightly golden, then return to baking dish. Bake in oven for about 30-40 minutes, or until internal thermometer reaches at least 165 degrees. Top with Bearnaise Sauce (p. 85) and serve.

Chicken Cordon Bleu Casserole 🍴 *(6-8 servings)*

1 cooked rotisserie chicken
2 (8 oz.) packages cubed ham
¼ cup butter
¼ cup gluten-free all-purpose flour (no XG)
2 cups whole milk
1 tbsp. Dijon mustard
1 tbsp. lemon juice

1 tsp. dried tarragon
¼ tsp. garlic powder
¼ tsp. sea salt
½ cup grated parmesan
2 cups grated Swiss cheese
1 cup gluten-free breadcrumbs
2 tbsp. butter, melted

Preheat oven to 350 degrees. Pull meat off the rotisserie chicken and lay in the bottom of a greased 9x13 inch baking dish, sprinkle cubed ham on top. In a medium saucepan, melt butter on medium heat. Whisk in flour and cook for 1 minute, then slowly add milk while constantly whisking. Add mustard, lemon juice, dried tarragon, garlic powder, and salt, whisk again. Cook for about 5 minutes, whisking constantly until sauce has thickened. Remove from heat and add parmesan cheese, stir until melted. Pour sauce evenly over chicken and ham in casserole dish. Sprinkle Swiss cheese on top, combine breadcrumbs and butter in a small bowl and toss together before sprinkling on top of Swiss cheese. Bake for 30 minutes, let sit for 5 minutes before serving. Serve over gluten-free pasta, rice, or mashed potatoes.

Chicken Croquettes 🍴 *(3 servings)*

2 (12.5 oz) cans white chicken meat
1 egg
1 tsp. Dijon mustard
¼ cup mayonnaise

¼ tsp. garlic powder
¼ tsp. onion powder
¼ tsp. black pepper
2/3 cup gluten-free breadcrumbs

Drain chicken very well in a colander, pushing down meat to squeeze out water. Preheat oven to 450 degrees. Combine all ingredients in a medium size mixing bowl and beat with electric mixer for about 1 minute, until everything is well-blended. Form into 6 hockey puck shaped patties and place on a pan in refrigerator for about 20 minutes. Remove from fridge, roll in more pork panko and bake for 15-18 minutes, or until lightly browned and crispy. Top with your choice of sauce (optional), serve on a bed of greens or with coleslaw.

This is like a land-lover version of Crab Cakes, just with chicken. Feel free to serve this with a Remoulade Sauce or Ranch Dressing with your Farm-Style Crab Cakes. The thought of anything Ranch with chicken just sounds like a match made in heaven.

Chicken Curry ♟ *(4 servings)*

For the Sauce
2 tbsp. olive oil
1 small yellow onion, diced
4 garlic cloves, minced
1 cup chicken broth
1 cup canned diced tomatoes, drained
Salt to taste
3 cups cooked chicken, diced
1 tsp. cornstarch
1/3 cup heavy cream

For the Spice Mix
1 tsp. ground ginger
1 ½ tsp. ground coriander
1 tsp. ground cumin
½ tsp. turmeric
½ tsp. fennel seeds
½ tsp. cinnamon
½ tsp. black pepper
¼ tsp. dry mustard
¼ tsp. ground cloves

Heat olive oil in a skillet on medium heat, add onion and sauté for about 5 minutes or until tender. Add garlic and sauté for 30 seconds, then add spice mix and sauté for another 30 seconds. Pour in chicken broth and diced tomatoes, bring to a boil then reduce heat to a simmer. Cover and cook for 5 minutes. Transfer mixture to a blender and puree until smooth, then return to skillet. Add salt and chicken, cover and cook until chicken is hot, about 5 minutes. Combine cornstarch with 2 teaspoons water, whisk together well before adding to sauce to thicken. Add heavy cream and stir, continue cooking for another 5 minutes for sauce to thicken. Serve over rice.

Chicken Divan ♟ *(6-8 servings)*

1 cup butter
½ cup gluten-free all-purpose flour (no XG)
½ cup cooking sherry or white wine
1 tbsp. onion powder
1 tsp. sea salt

2 tsp. chicken bouillon
4 cups whole milk
1 ½ lbs. cooked chicken, diced
1 ½ lbs. broccoli florets
2 cups grated cheddar cheese

Preheat oven to 350 degrees. In a large pot, fill halfway with water and bring to a boil on medium/high heat. Dump broccoli florets into pot and cook for about 3 minutes. Pour broccoli into a strainer to drain completely and set aside. Melt butter in a pot on medium heat. Whisk in flour, salt, and chicken bouillon, cook for another minute. Slowly whisk in milk, continue cooking for about 10 minutes for sauce to thicken. Evenly distribute chicken and broccoli florets in a greased 9x13 inch baking dish, pour sauce to evenly coat the meat and veggies. Don't be shy, they love to be smothered with this heavenly sauce. Sprinkle grated cheese on top. Bake in oven for 35-45 minutes, or until hot. Serve with rice, mashed potatoes, gluten-free pasta or more veggies.

Chicken Fricassee 🍴 *(4-6 servings)*

1 tbsp. olive oil
8 chicken thighs and legs
Salt and pepper to taste
1 tbsp. butter
1 small onion, chopped
2 cloves garlic, minced

2 medium carrots, peeled and sliced
1 tsp. dried thyme
2 tbsp. gluten-free all-purpose flour (no XG)
½ cup dry white wine
1 ½ cups chicken broth
½ cup heavy cream

Preheat oven to 350 degrees. Using a paper towel, pat chicken dry and season with salt and pepper. Bring a large deep pan over medium heat with 1 tablespoon olive oil. Cook chicken for about 4 minutes on each side, until golden but not cooked through. Remove chicken to a plate and set aside. Leave about 1 tablespoon of excess fat in pan, add butter, onions and carrots. Cook on low heat for about 8-10 minutes, add garlic and thyme, cook for 30 seconds. Add flour and cook, stirring until flour is absorbed by the fat. Add white wine and simmer until slightly reduced, then pour in chicken broth. Return chicken to the pan, then place in oven and bake for about 45 minutes or until chicken reaches internal temperature of 165 degrees. Remove from oven, add heavy cream and stir. Season with more salt and pepper if desired, serve warm.

Chicken Jalfrezi 🍴 *(4 servings)*

3 (5 oz.) chicken breasts, diced
1 tsp. ground cumin
1 tsp. ground coriander
1 tsp. turmeric
¼ cup olive oil, divided
1 large onion, divided
2 cloves garlic, minced
1 green chili, minced

14 oz. can plum tomatoes
1 tbsp. ground coriander
1 tbsp. ground cumin
1 tsp. turmeric
1 red bell pepper, seeded and diced
2 red chilies, diced
2 tsp. garam masala

Combine diced chicken breasts and 1 tsp. cumin, 1 tsp. coriander, and 1 tsp. turmeric, toss together, leave in refrigerator to marinate while making the sauce. Pour 2 tbsp. olive oil in a skillet on medium heat, dice ½ of onion and sauté until browned, about 5 minutes. Add garlic and green chili, continue cooking for another minute. Add 1 ¼ cups water, simmer for about 20 minutes. Spoon plum tomatoes into a food processor and puree until smooth. In another pan, add 1 tbsp. olive oil, 1 tbsp. ground coriander, 1 tbsp. ground cumin, and 1 tsp. turmeric. Sauté for one minute, then add tomatoes to the pan and simmer for about ten minutes. Pour onion mixture into food processor or blender and puree until smooth, then add to pan with tomatoes and simmer for 20 minutes. Add remaining 1 tbsp. olive oil to the pan you cooked the onion mixture in, then sauté chicken until lightly browned. Slice remaining ½ onion and add to pan with chicken along with red bell pepper and red chilies, cook until the vegetables soften. Add sauce to chicken, simmer for 10-15 minutes, adding water if it gets too thick. Just before serving, add garam masala and stir, serve warm with rice.

Chicken Marbella 🍴 *(6 servings)*

1 whole chicken, cut up
3 bay leaves
1 head garlic, peeled
½ cup pitted prunes
½ cup pitted green olives
¼ cup capers

¼ cup red wine vinegar
¼ cup olive oil
2 tbsp. dried oregano
Salt and pepper, to taste
½ cup white wine
½ cup light brown sugar

In a large mixing bowl, combine bay leaves, garlic, prunes, olives, capers, red wine vinegar, olive oil, oregano, salt, and pepper. Stir together until combined, then add chicken and push it all together. Lift the skin of the chicken so the marinade hangs on the flesh of the chicken. Cover bowl and set in refrigerator overnight to marinate. The next day, preheat oven to 350 degrees. Pour the chicken and marinade (including prunes, olives, garlic, etc.) into a large baking dish and spread it out into one even layer so the chicken is not overlapping. Pour white wine into baking dish and sprinkle with brown sugar. Place dish in oven and bake for 50-60 minutes, basting with the pan juices a few times during the cooking process. When the chicken reaches an internal temperature of 165 degrees, remove dish from oven and transfer chicken to a large serving platter. Spoon the prunes, olives, and capers on top. Pour the juices from the roasting pan into a saucepan and bring to a boil over medium heat until the sauce reduces to about half the amount. Strain sauce into a bowl, then pour over chicken and serve warm.

Chicken Marsala 🍴 *(6-8 servings)*

1 cup butter
½ cup gluten-free all-purpose flour (no XG)
1 tbsp. minced garlic
1 cup marsala cooking wine
2 cups chicken broth
1 cup heavy cream
½ tsp. black pepper

1 ½ tsp. sea salt
½ cup grated parmesan
1 lb. gluten-free penne pasta
1 lb. cooked chicken, diced
6 oz. mushrooms, sliced
1 lb. grated mozzarella cheese

Preheat oven to 350 degrees. Melt butter in a pot on medium heat. Whisk in flour and cook for another minute, add garlic and stir. Slowly whisk in marsala, followed by chicken broth, then heavy cream. Continue cooking for about 10 minutes for sauce to thicken, stirring occasionally. Meanwhile, cook pasta according to package directions for al dente and drain. In another pan, sauté mushrooms in 1 tablespoon olive oil until tender, drain and set aside. When sauce has thickened, stir in salt, pepper, and parmesan until cheese is melted and smooth. Remove from heat, stir in chicken, mushrooms, and cooked pasta. Spoon evenly into a greased 9x13 inch baking dish, top with mozzarella. Bake in oven for 25-30 minutes, or until hot.

Chicken Nuggets *(3-4 servings)*

1 lb. ground chicken
2 tbsp. milk
½ cup gluten-free breadcrumbs
1 egg, beaten
¾ tsp. garlic salt
¼ cup grated parmesan cheese

Preheat oven to 375 degrees. Combine all ingredients in a medium size mixing bowl and mix well using hands. Scoop 2 tablespoons of mixture out at a time to create little nuggets, lay on a greased baking pan. Place pan in oven to bake for 8 minutes, then flip nuggets over to continue baking for another 8 minutes. Serve warm.

Chicken Parmesan *(4 servings)*

4 (5 oz.) boneless skinless chicken breasts
2 large eggs
1 cup gluten-free all-purpose flour
1 cup gluten-free panko breadcrumbs
¾ cup grated parmesan, divided
½ cup olive oil
24 oz. jar gluten-free spaghetti sauce
1 cup grated mozzarella cheese

Preheat oven to 350 degrees. Lay one chicken breast between 2 pieces of plastic wrap, pound to ½ inch thick. Repeat process with other chicken breasts. Beat eggs with 2 tablespoons water in a wide, shallow bowl, set aside. Place flour in another shallow bowl, and in a third shallow bowl toss together breadcrumbs and ½ cup grated parmesan. Dredge each side of each piece of chicken in flour, followed by egg mixture, then breadcrumb mixture. Set aside on a plate. Heat olive oil in a skillet pan on medium heat, fry each piece of chicken on each side for about 3 minutes, until golden. Place in a greased 9x13 inch baking dish. Pour spaghetti sauce on top of chicken, followed by remaining parmesan. Sprinkle mozzarella on top and bake in oven for about 20-25 minutes, until chicken is no longer pink in the center. Serve with pasta or vegetables.

Chicken Parmesan Casserole *(4-6 servings)*

2 cups cooked chicken, diced
24 oz. jar gluten-free spaghetti sauce
½ cup grated Parmesan cheese
2 cups grated mozzarella cheese
½ cup breadcrumbs
4 tbsp. butter, melted

Preheat oven to 375 degrees. Spread chicken into the bottom of an 8x8 inch baking dish. Pour spaghetti sauce on top of chicken into an even layer, making sure all the chicken is completely covered. Sprinkle Parmesan cheese on top of sauce, followed by mozzarella cheese. Sprinkle breadcrumbs on top of mozzarella, drizzle melted butter on top of breadcrumbs. Bake for 30 minutes. Serve hot with cooked pasta or veggies.

Chicken Piccata *(4 servings)*

4 (5 oz.) boneless, skinless chicken breasts
Salt and pepper to taste
Gluten-free all-purpose flour (as needed)
6 tbsp. unsalted butter
5 tbsp. olive oil
1/3 cup lemon juice
2 cups chicken broth
¼ cup brined capers, rinsed
2 tbsp. fresh parsley, chopped

Season chicken with salt and pepper. Dredge chicken in flour and shake off excess. In a large skillet over medium high heat, melt 2 tablespoons butter with olive oil. When butter and oil start to sizzle, add 2 pieces of chicken and cook for 3 minutes. When chicken is browned, flip and cook other side for 3 minutes. Remove and transfer to plate. Remove pan from heat. Into the pan add the lemon juice, stock and capers. Return to stove and bring to boil, scraping up brown bits from the pan for extra flavor. Return all the chicken to the pan, cover and simmer for about 5-10 minutes until fully cooked. Remove chicken to platter. Add remaining 2 tablespoons butter to sauce and whisk vigorously. Pour sauce over chicken and garnish with parsley.

Chicken Pot Pie *(6-8 servings)*

1 lb. butter
1 cup gluten-free all-purpose flour (no XG)
1 tbsp. chicken bouillon
1 ½ tbsp. onion powder
5 cups whole milk
2 tsp. sea salt
½ tsp. black pepper
2 ½ lbs. cooked chicken, diced
24 oz. frozen mixed veggies, thawed
Savory Pie Crust (p. 222)

Preheat oven to 350 degrees. Melt butter in a pot on medium heat. Whisk in flour and cook for another minute, add chicken bouillon and onion powder, stir. Slowly whisk in milk, continue cooking for about 10 minutes to allow sauce to thicken. When sauce has thickened, stir in salt and pepper. Remove from heat, stir in chicken and veggies, and spoon into a greased 9x13 inch baking dish. Shape and roll pie crust to ¼ inch thick to cover filling, lay on top. Bake in oven for 35-45 minutes, until hot and crust is golden brown. Let sit for five minutes before serving.

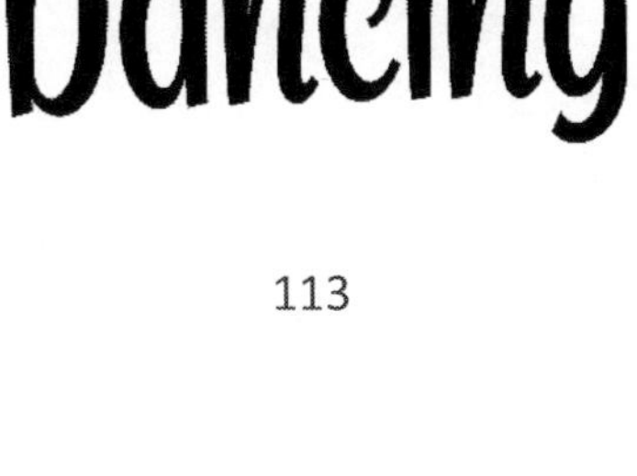

Chicken Sauté 🍴 *(4 servings)*

4 (5 oz.) boneless chicken breasts
2 tsp. garlic powder
2 tsp. onion powder
2 tsp. Italian seasoning

1 tsp. paprika
1 tsp. sea salt
½ tsp. black pepper
3 tbsp. olive oil, divided

Make sure each chicken breast has an equal thickness throughout each piece. You can do this by placing a piece of plastic wrap over each piece and pounding down the thicker parts using the flat part of a meat mallet. In a small bowl, whisk together garlic powder, onion powder, Italian seasoning, paprika, salt, and pepper. Drizzle 1 tablespoon olive oil over chicken breasts, then generously rub seasoning all over each side. Heat a large skillet on medium/high heat and add remaining 2 tablespoons olive oil. Add chicken breasts to pan and cook for about 5 minutes on each side. Decrease heat if it gets too hot and starts spitting at you. When the chicken has browned on both sides, check the internal temperature to make sure it has reached 165 degrees. Remove chicken from pan, set aside to rest for 2-3 minutes before serving over salad or with your favorite side dishes.

Chicken Shawarma 🍴🍴 *(6 servings)*

2 tsp. ground cumin
2 tsp. turmeric powder
2 tsp. ground coriander
2 tsp. garlic powder
2 tsp. paprika
½ tsp. ground cloves
¼ tsp. cayenne
½ tsp. salt

8 boneless, skinless chicken thighs
1 large onion, thinly sliced
1 large lemon, juiced
1/3 cup olive oil
6 pieces gluten-free pita bread
Lemon Tahini Dressing (p. 98)
Baby Arugula

Combine cumin, turmeric, coriander, garlic powder, paprika, cloves, and cayenne in a small bowl and whisk together, set aside. Pat the chicken thighs dry with a paper towel, season with salt on both sides and cut into bite-size pieces. In a medium size mixing bowl, combine chicken, seasoning mix, lemon juice, and olive oil. Toss together, cover and refrigerate for a minimum of 3 hours or overnight. When ready to eat, remove chicken from refrigerator and preheat oven to 425 degrees. Grease a sheet pan with cooking spray, then spread chicken mixture into an even layer. Roast for 30 minutes in oven. While chicken is cooking, slice each pita bread to make pita pockets, and make Lemon Tahini Dressing (p. 98). To serve, slice open pita pockets, stuff with chicken, arugula, and drizzle with dressing. Serve warm.

Chicken Tikka Masala 🍴 *(4-6 servings)*

3 boneless, skinless chicken breasts
½ cup plain yogurt
2 tbsp. lemon juice
6 garlic cloves, minced
1 tbsp. minced ginger
2 tsp. salt
2 tsp. ground cumin
2 tsp. garam masala
2 tsp. paprika
3 tbsp. olive oil
1 large onion, diced

2 tbsp. minced ginger
8 garlic cloves, minced
2 tsp. ground cumin
2 tsp. ground turmeric
2 tsp. ground coriander
2 tsp. paprika
2 tsp. chili powder
2 tsp. garam masala
3 ½ cups tomato sauce
1 ¼ cups water
1 cup heavy cream

Cut chicken into bite size chunks and place in a medium size mixing bowl. Add yogurt, lemon juice, 6 garlic cloves, 1 tbsp. ginger, salt, 2 tsp. cumin, 2 tsp. garam masala, and 2 tsp. paprika, stir together well. Cover and refrigerate for at least one hour or overnight. When ready to eat, preheat oven to 500 degrees. Using a high-sided baking pan or roasted pan, line bottom with parchment paper. Slide each piece of marinated chicken on bamboo or wooden skewers, leaving enough room on each end to set on edges of pan to keep chicken elevated for even roasting. Bake for about 15 minutes, until slightly dark brown. While the chicken is cooking, prepare sauce. Heat olive oil in a large pot over medium heat, add onions and sauté for about 5 minutes. Add ginger and garlic, cook for another minute. Add remaining cumin, turmeric, coriander, paprika, chili powder, and garam masala, stir constantly for about 30 seconds. Add tomato sauce and water, stir together well and bring to a boil, cook for about 5 minutes. Add heavy cream and stir, then remove cooked chicken from skewers and add to sauce. Cook for another two minutes before serving hot with rice.

Chicken Tetrazzini 🍴 *(6-8 servings)*

1 cup butter
½ cup gluten-free all-purpose flour (no XG)
2 cups chicken broth
2 cups milk
½ cup freshly grated parmesan

1 ½ teaspoons salt
1 lb. gluten-free spaghetti
1 lb. cooked chicken, diced
2 cups grated mozzarella

Preheat oven to 350 degrees. Melt butter in a pot on medium heat. Whisk in flour and cook for another minute. Slowly whisk in milk and chicken broth, continue cooking for about 10 minutes to allow sauce to thicken. Meanwhile, cook pasta according to package directions for al dente and drain. When sauce has thickened, stir in salt and parmesan until cheese is melted and smooth. Remove from heat, stir in chicken and cooked pasta. Spoon into greased 9x13 inch baking dish, top with mozzarella. Bake in oven for 25-30 minutes, until hot and cheese is melted.

Chicken Zucchini Casserole 🍴 *(4 servings)*

8 oz. mushrooms
2 medium zucchini
¼ cup butter
Salt and pepper, to taste
4 cups grated Italian cheese blend, divided

8 oz. sour cream
4 green onions, sliced
4 eggs, beaten
1 tbsp. Italian seasoning
1 lb. cooked chicken, diced

Preheat oven to 375 degrees. Wipe mushrooms clean with a damp paper towel, remove stems and slice into ¼ inch thick pieces. Slice zucchini into ¼ inch thick halves or quarters. Melt butter in a large pan on medium heat, add mushrooms and zucchini, cook for about five minutes or until tender. Drain in a colander. In a medium size mixing bowl, combine sour cream, 2 cups cheese, green onions, eggs, Italian seasoning, salt and pepper. Stir together well, then add drained vegetables and diced chicken. Spread into a greased 8x8 inch baking dish, top with remaining 2 cups of cheese. Bake for 30-35 minutes, remove dish from oven and let cool for about 5 minutes before serving.

Chipotle Chicken Thighs 🍴 *(4 servings)*

1 lb. boneless chicken thighs
Salt and pepper to taste

1 can chipotle peppers in adobo sauce
2 tbsp. olive oil

Lay chicken thighs on a cutting board and season with salt and pepper on both sides, then transfer to a gallon size freezer bag. Finely dice chipotle peppers in sauce, spoon into bag with chicken. Seal the bag and mix until the chicken is fully coated, marinate for a minimum of two hours or overnight. Heat oil in a large skillet on medium heat, cook chicken until golden brown, about 4 minutes on each side or until internal temperature reaches 165 degrees. Serve warm.

Cilantro Lime Chicken 🍴 *(6 servings)*

3 tbsp. olive oil, divided
2 limes, juiced and zested
3 cloves garlic, minced
1 tbsp. honey
1 tsp. ground cumin

½ tsp. chili powder
1 tsp. salt
½ tsp. black pepper
6 boneless chicken thighs
¼ cup chopped cilantro leaves

Combine 2 tablespoons olive oil, juice and zest from limes, garlic, honey, cumin, chili powder, salt, and pepper in a medium size mixing bowl and whisk together well. Add chicken thighs, cover with sauce and marinate for at least one hour. Preheat oven to 400 degrees. Heat remaining 1 tbsp. olive oil in a skillet over medium/high heat. Sear the chicken on both sides for about 2 minutes before transferring to a greased 9x13 inch baking dish. Bake for 15-20 minutes or until internal temperature reaches 165 degrees. Let cool for 5 minutes before serving, garnish with cilantro leaves.

Country Fried Chicken Breasts 🍴 *(6 servings)*

6 (5 oz.) boneless chicken breasts
1 cup gluten-free all-purpose flour
1 cup gluten-free cornmeal
2 tsp. baking powder
1 tsp. baking soda
1 tsp. salt

1 tsp. black pepper
1 tsp. garlic powder
1 ½ cups buttermilk
1 egg
1 tbsp. hot sauce
Oil, for frying

Cover chicken breasts with plastic wrap and pound the thick parts down so the chicken has even layers of thickness. In a medium size mixing bowl, combine flour, cornmeal, baking powder, baking soda, salt, pepper, and garlic powder, whisk together well. In another bowl, combine buttermilk, egg, and hot sauce, whisk together well. Dredge chicken in flour mixture, then buttermilk mixture, then back to the flour mixture for a second time to make sure each piece is covered well. Heat oil in a deep fryer or large skillet (at least 2 inches deep) on medium heat or to 350 degrees. Fry chicken breasts on each side for 4-5 minutes, until golden brown and cooked through. Transfer to a plate lined with paper towels to catch excess grease. Serve warm with Country Gravy (p. 86).

Creamed Chicken and Biscuits 🍴 *(4-6 servings)*

¼ cup butter
¼ cup gluten-free all-purpose flour (no XG)
2 cups milk
1 tsp. chicken bouillon

½ teaspoon onion powder
1 cooked rotisserie chicken
Buttermilk Biscuits (p. 49)

Pick meat off rotisserie chicken and set aside. Melt butter in a medium saucepan on medium heat. Whisk in flour; continue to cook for another minute, whisking constantly. Slowly add milk and continue to stir. Add chicken bouillon and onion powder, continue to stir and cook on medium heat for another minute. Reduce heat to low-medium, continue to cook and stir constantly. When sauce thickens, add chicken. Split biscuits into two pieces, place on plates. Spoon sauce over biscuits and serve warm.

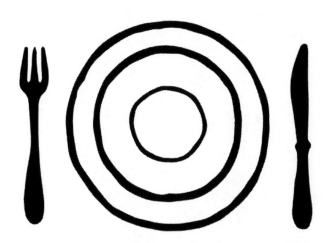

117

Creamy Chicken and Rice 🍴 *(8-10 servings)*

1 cup butter
½ cup gluten-free all-purpose flour (no XG)
2 (1 oz.) ranch dressing packets
6 cups whole milk
2 cups chicken broth
1 tsp. salt

½ tsp. pepper
2 lbs. cooked chicken, diced
2 cups uncooked rice + 4 cups water
24 oz. frozen mixed vegetables
2 cups gluten-free breadcrumbs
½ cup butter, melted

Preheat oven to 350 degrees. Melt butter in a pot on medium heat. Whisk in flour and ranch dressing packets, cook for another minute. Slowly whisk in milk and chicken broth, continue cooking for about 10 minutes to allow sauce to thicken. While sauce is cooking, cook rice according to package directions in a separate pot. When sauce has thickened, stir in salt and pepper. Remove from heat, stir in chicken, rice, and veggies, distribute evenly into a greased 9x13 inch baking dish. In a small mixing bowl, toss together breadcrumbs and melted butter, sprinkle on top. Bake in oven for 35-45 minutes, until hot and topping is golden brown.

The sauce will seem thin when you make this compared to other sauce recipes in this book, which is normal. The sauce will soak into the rice and will thicken during the baking process, so it won't actually be like eating soup. Promise.

Crunchy Lemon Chicken 🍴 *(4 servings)*

4 (5 oz.) chicken breasts
2 cups crushed gluten-free corn flakes
2 tbsp. lemon-pepper seasoning
¼ tsp. salt

¼ tsp. black pepper
¼ cup butter, melted
¼ cup lemon juice
1 tbsp. lemon zest

Preheat oven to 375 degrees. Cover chicken breasts with plastic wrap and pound the thick parts down so each piece has an even layer of thickness. Combine corn flakes, lemon-pepper seasoning, salt, and pepper in a shallow bowl and toss together. In another shallow bowl, combine melted butter, lemon juice, and lemon zest, whisk together well. Dip each piece of chicken in the butter mixture, then into the corn flake mixture to coat completely on both sides. Lay each piece of chicken in a greased 9x13 inch baking dish, bake for about 25 minutes or until internal temperature reaches 165 degrees. Serve warm.

Garlic Chicken ↑ *(4-6 servings)*

3 large boneless chicken breasts
2 tbsp. gluten-free all-purpose flour (no XG)
½ tsp. salt
½ tsp. black pepper
2 tbsp. olive oil

1 tbsp. minced garlic
3 tbsp. chopped fresh parsley
3 tbsp. butter, divided
1 cup chicken broth

Cut chicken into 1-inch cubes and pat dry with a paper towel. Combine with 1 tbsp. flour, salt, and pepper in a bowl, toss together well. Heat 2 tbsp. olive oil in a large skillet on medium heat. Cook chicken in skillet in one layer for 4-5 minutes, then turn over and continue cooking for another 4-5 minutes until it develops a golden crust. Combine garlic and parsley in a small bowl and toss together. Add 2 tbsp. butter to the pan along with garlic and parsley and stir, sauté for about one minute. Using a spoon, transfer chicken to a plate and set aside. Add remaining 1 tbsp. butter to pan. When butter has melted, add remaining 1 tbsp. flour and whisk constantly for about one minute. Slowly whisk in chicken broth, continue cooking while stirring constantly until gravy has thickened. Return chicken to pan to coat with gravy and serve warm.

Ginger Chicken ↑↑ *(4-6 servings)*

2 eggs + 2 tbsp. water
¾ cup gluten-free all-purpose flour
2 tbsp. cornstarch
1 tsp. garlic powder
1 tsp. ground ginger
1 tsp. paprika
1 tsp. salt
½ tsp. black pepper
1 ½ lbs. chicken tenders
Oil, for frying

½ tsp. red pepper flakes
½ cup gluten-free soy sauce
1 tbsp. sriracha
1 tsp. fresh ginger, minced
3 garlic cloves, minced
½ tsp. black pepper
2 tbsp. honey
1 tbsp. sesame seeds
2 green onions, chopped

Whisk the eggs in a shallow bowl and set aside. In another shallow bowl, combine flour, cornstarch, garlic powder, ground ginger, paprika, salt, and ½ tsp. black pepper, whisk together well to combine. Dip each chicken finger in eggs, then dredge in flour mixture. Fill a Dutch oven or large pan with at least 2 inches of oil, fry chicken tenders a few at a time for 4-5 minutes or until they're golden brown and fully cooked. Repeat process until all chicken tenders are cooked, lay on plate lined with paper towels to drain excess grease. In a small mixing bowl, combine red pepper flakes, soy sauce, sriracha, fresh ginger, garlic cloves, black pepper, and honey, whisk together well. Transfer chicken tenders to a serving plate or platter, drizzle with sauce and sprinkle with sesame seeds and green onions before serving.

Grilled Chicken Breasts ⸸ *(4 servings)*

4 boneless chicken breasts
6 tbsp. olive oil
4 garlic cloves, minced
1 tsp. dried thyme

½ tsp. dried oregano
1 tsp. salt
½ tsp. black pepper
Juice and zest from 1 lemon

Place a piece of plastic wrap over each chicken breast and pound to an even ½ inch thickness. Transfer chicken to a gallon size freezer bag. In a small mixing bowl, whisk together olive oil, garlic, thyme, oregano, salt, pepper, lemon juice and zest. Pour into bag with chicken breasts, seal and massage together to make sure chicken is completely coated in marinade. Place in refrigerator for at least 4 hours. Preheat grill to high heat, oil the grates and cook chicken for about 3-4 minutes on each side, until internal temperature reaches 165 degrees.

Grilled Chicken Thighs ⸸ *(6-8 servings)*

½ cup light brown sugar
¼ cup paprika
1 tsp. black pepper
3 tsp. salt
2 tsp. garlic powder

2 tsp. onion powder
½ tsp. cayenne
2 lbs. boneless chicken thighs
½ cup gluten-free BBQ sauce

In a small mixing bowl, combine brown sugar, paprika, pepper, salt, garlic powder, onion powder, and cayenne, whisk together well. Generously rub all over both sides of chicken thighs and set aside. Preheat grill to high heat, oil the grates and cook chicken for about 5-6 minutes on each side, or until internal temperature reaches 165 degrees. Brush with BBQ sauce and serve warm.

Hawaiian Chicken ⸸ *(10-12 servings)*

4 lbs. boneless chicken thighs
1 cup pineapple juice
¾ cup light brown sugar

¼ cup gluten-free teriyaki sauce
¼ cup gluten-free soy sauce
1 lb. smoked sausage

Lay chicken thighs in a slow cooker. Whisk together pineapple juice, brown sugar, teriyaki sauce and soy sauce in a small mixing bowl, pour over chicken. Cook on low for 3 hours. Slice sausage into ¼ inch rounds. Shred chicken, add sausage, and cook on low for 1 more hour. Serve warm with Buttered Rice (p. 184) and Green Beans (p. 188).

⸸**Pro-Tip:** feel free to mix up the boneless chicken thighs with boneless chicken breasts for a variety of light and dark meat.

Herb-Roasted Chicken ♔ *(6-8 servings)*

¼ cup butter, softened
4 whole garlic cloves, 1 minced garlic clove
½ tsp. dried rosemary
½ tsp. dried thyme
Salt and pepper

4 lb. whole chicken, giblets removed
1 large onion, cut into 8 chunks
1 lemon, zested and sliced
1 cup chicken broth

Preheat oven to 425 degrees, position rack in the lower third of the oven. In a small bowl, combine butter, minced garlic, zest of lemon, dried rosemary and thyme, stir together well. Rub half of butter mixture under the skin of the chicken, and the rest all over the outside. Season with salt and pepper. Lay the chicken breast side up on the rack of a roasting pan. Spread the onion chunks, lemon slices, whole garlic cloves, and ½ cup water in the bottom of the pan under the rack. Roast chicken in oven for 30 minutes, until the breast is just starting to lightly brown in spots. Turn chicken breast-side-down using tongs, roast for another 20 minutes. Turn the chicken back to breast-side-up and pour another ½ cup of water in the pan, roast for another 20 minutes or until a thermometer inserted in the inner thigh registers 175-180 degrees. Tilt the chicken to drain juices into pan, then transfer to a cutting board. Remove rack from pan, spoon fat off the top. Set pan over high heat on stove, add stock and cook. Scrape up any browned bits and press lemon slices to release juices into the gravy. Cook until reduced, about 5 minutes. Pour through a strainer and serve gravy on the side, carve chicken and serve.

Honey Mustard Chicken Tenders ♔ *(4-6 servings)*

2 lbs. boneless, skinless chicken tenders
½ cup Dijon mustard

½ cup honey
¼ cup butter, melted

In a small bowl, whisk together mustard, honey, and melted butter. Place chicken in a zipper gallon freezer bag, pour liquid into bag. Seal bag and place in the refrigerator for the chicken to marinate for at least 1 hour. Preheat the oven to 350 degrees, remove chicken from refrigerator and pour into 9x13 inch baking dish. Place in oven and bake for about 20 minutes, or until thermometer reads at least 165 degrees. Serve warm.

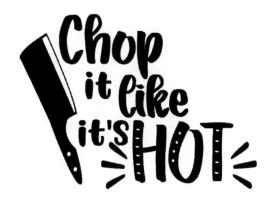

Jamaican Jerk Chicken 🍴 *(8-10 servings)*

One whole cut-up chicken
1/3 cup olive oil
2 tbsp. light brown sugar
1 tbsp. dried thyme
2 tsp. ground allspice
2 tsp. paprika
½ tsp. ground cinnamon

1 tsp. ground ginger
1 tsp. ground cloves
½ tsp. cayenne
1 tsp. garlic powder
1 tsp. onion powder
2 tsp. salt
¼ tsp. black pepper

Preheat oven to 425 degrees. Pat chicken pieces dry using a paper towel. In a small mixing bowl, combine all remaining ingredients and mix into a paste. Generously rub paste all over each piece of chicken, place on a foil-lined baking sheet with space in between each piece. Place pan in oven to bake for 45-50 minutes, or until an internal thermometer reads 165 degrees in the largest piece of chicken. Serve immediately with drippings from pan.

Korean BBQ Chicken 🍴 *(4-6 servings)*

1/3 cup gluten-free soy sauce
2 tbsp. ketchup
½ tsp. cumin
½ tsp. garlic powder
1 tsp. paprika
½ tsp. ground ginger
1 tbsp. rice wine vinegar
1 tbsp. honey

2 tbsp. light brown sugar
2 tsp. sriracha
1/3 cup chicken broth
1 tbsp. cornstarch
2 tbsp. sesame oil
2 lbs. boneless chicken breasts
2 tbsp. sesame seeds
2 green onions, sliced

In a small mixing bowl, combine soy sauce, ketchup, cumin, garlic powder, paprika, ginger, rice wine vinegar, honey, brown sugar, and sriracha, whisk together well. Combine chicken broth and cornstarch, whisk together until cornstarch has dissolved. Cut chicken into 1-inch chunks and set aside. Heat sesame oil in a large skillet over medium heat. Add chicken to skillet and cook for about 5 minutes, until white on the outside but not fully cooked through. Add sauce mixture to the skillet, stir to coat and cook for about 3 minutes. Pour broth and cornstarch in pan, continue cooking for another 4-6 minutes or until chicken is fully cooked through and the sauce has thickened. When ready to serve, sprinkle with sesame seeds and sliced green onions. Serve warm with Fried Rice (p. 188).

Lemon Chicken ♦ *(4-6 servings)*

2 large boneless chicken breasts
1 tbsp. gluten-free soy sauce
1 tbsp. white wine
¼ cup gluten-free cornstarch
¼ cup gluten-free all-purpose flour
Oil, for frying

3 tbsp. lemon juice
1 tbsp. granulated sugar
5 tbsp. water
1 tbsp. gluten-free cornstarch
¼ tsp. salt
1 tsp. white sesame seeds

Slice chicken breasts into bite-size chunks and place in a large freezer bag with soy sauce and white wine. Close bag and make sure all chicken is coated, marinate for at least 30 minutes. In a small bowl, whisk together cornstarch and all-purpose flour, then add to bag with chicken and shake very well so that all chicken is coated evenly. Pour enough oil in a large pot or skillet so that it's about 2 inches deep, heat on medium high or use a deep fryer at 350 degrees. When oil is hot, fry chicken pieces until golden brown, transfer to a plate lined with paper towels to soak up excess grease. In a small saucepan, combine lemon juice, granulated sugar, water, 1 tbsp. cornstarch and salt. Bring to a quick boil, stirring often until slightly thickened. Transfer chicken to a serving bowl, pour sauce on top and toss together. Sprinkle with sesame seeds and serve.

Margarita Chicken ♦ *(10-12 servings)*

4 lbs. boneless, skinless chicken breasts
2 tbsp. minced garlic
1 tbsp. onion powder
2 tsp. salt
2 tsp. black pepper

1 ½ cups margarita mix
½ cup tequila
½ cup triple sec
¼ cup honey
1 ½ cups extra-virgin olive oil

Place chicken breasts in freezer bags. Combine garlic, onion powder, salt, pepper, margarita mix, tequila, triple sec, honey, and oil in a blender and puree until smooth. Pour marinade equally between bags and seal tightly. Squeeze gently to make sure all the chicken is coated in sauce. When ready to cook, dump ingredients into a slow cooker and cook on low for 4 hours or until chicken is cooked through (at least 165 degrees). Shred chicken using two forks, serve warm with Mexican Rice (p. 190), tacos, fajitas, or burritos.

♦ **Pro-Tip:** feel free to mix up the boneless chicken breasts with boneless chicken thighs for a variety of light and dark meat.

Moroccan Chicken ♔ *(4-6 servings)*

1 tsp. paprika	Salt and pepper to taste
1 tsp. ground cumin	2 tbsp. olive oil
¼ tsp. cayenne	1 large onion, cut into ¼ inch pieces
½ tsp. ground ginger	2 tbsp. gluten-free all-purpose flour (no XG)
½ tsp. ground coriander	1 ½ cups chicken broth
¼ tsp. ground cinnamon	2 tbsp. honey
1 lemon, zested and juiced	3 medium carrots, peeled
5 garlic cloves, minced	½ cup green olives
4 lbs. chicken thighs	2 tbsp. chopped fresh cilantro

In a small bowl, combine paprika, cumin, cayenne, ginger, coriander, and cinnamon, stir together and set aside. Combine lemon zest and garlic, set aside. Season chicken on both sides with salt and pepper. Heat oil in a large pan over medium/high heat. When oil is hot, brown chicken pieces in a single layer on each side until a deep golden color, about 5 minutes per side. Transfer chicken to a large plate. Reduce heat to medium, add onion and cook until tender, about 5 minutes. Add lemon zest and garlic, stirring for 30 seconds until fragrant. Add spices that were set aside along with flour, stir constantly and cook for about 30 seconds. Add broth and honey, scraping the bottom of the pan to loosen any browned bits. Add the chicken back to the pan, reduce heat to medium/low, cover and simmer for 10 minutes. While chicken is cooking, slice peeled carrots into ½ inch thick circles, add to the pan and cook while covered for another 10 minutes or until tender. Stir in olives and cilantro, serve immediately.

Nacho Baked Chicken ♗ *(6 servings)*

6 (5 oz.) boneless, skinless chicken breasts	1 tsp. seasoned salt
1 cup mayonnaise	1 bag gluten-free cheddar nachos*

In food processor or food chopper, crush all chips to a fine consistency, set aside in a shallow bowl. In another small bowl, whisk seasoned salt with mayonnaise. One chicken breast at a time, brush one side with mayonnaise, dredge in chips. Coat other side with mayonnaise, turn over and press into chips. Repeat until all chicken breasts are coated with crushed chips. Place chicken in a greased 9x13 inch baking dish and bake in oven for approximately 30 minutes, or until chicken reaches 165 degrees internally. Serve warm.

Pro-Tip: A great brand of chips for this recipe that are certified gluten-free is Simply Organic Gluten-Free White Cheddar Doritos®! The classic Doritos® doesn't contain gluten ingredients, but they are not certified gluten-free. If you get a knock-off brand, be sure to check the label to see what ingredients are used.

Pan-Fried Chicken 🍴 *(4-6 servings)*

8 pieces of chicken (drumsticks or thighs)
3 cups buttermilk
1 ½ cups gluten-free all-purpose flour

2 tsp. salt
1 tsp. black pepper
½ tsp. cayenne

In a large bowl, combine chicken and buttermilk, toss together to make sure all chicken pieces are covered by the buttermilk. Cover with plastic wrap, place in refrigerator to marinate for a minimum of 8 hours or overnight. When ready to cook chicken, combine flour, salt, pepper, and cayenne in a large resealable freezer bag and toss together to combine will. Place two cooling racks over rimmed baking sheets. Pull each piece of chicken out of the buttermilk and scrape off most of the liquid against the side of the bowl, then add to bag with flour mixture. Do this a few pieces of chicken at a time, shake bag to coat completely. Transfer chicken pieces to racks and press flour to help it stick to the chicken as you remove it from the bag. Pour at least 2 inches oil into a large skillet, heat to 350 degrees. Add chicken pieces to oil, making sure you do not crowd the skillet. Fry until the chicken is golden, crisp, and cooked through, which will take about 20-25 minutes. Turn chicken over halfway through cooking process, make sure internal temperature reaches 165 degrees. Line racks with paper towels and set cooked chicken pieces on top to drain. Serve warm.

Paprika Chicken 🍴 *(4 servings)*

2 large boneless chicken breasts
2 tsp. paprika
1 tsp. poultry seasoning
1 tsp. salt

½ tsp. black pepper
2 tbsp. olive oil
1 lemon, juiced

Cut chicken breasts into 1-inch cubes and place in a small mixing bowl. In another small bowl, whisk together paprika, poultry seasoning, salt, and pepper. Sprinkle over chicken cubes and toss to combine. Heat olive oil on medium heat in a skillet, add chicken and sauté on one side for 5 minutes. Turn pieces over and cook for another 3-4 minutes or until cooked through. Drizzle with lemon juice and serve warm.

Parmesan Chicken Tenders 🍴 *(4-6 servings)*

2 lbs. boneless chicken tenders
½ cup mayonnaise

1 tsp. Italian seasoning
½ cup grated parmesan cheese

Preheat oven to 350 degrees. Lay chicken tenders in a greased 9x13 inch baking dish. Brush mayonnaise evenly on top of tenders, sprinkle with parmesan cheese then Italian seasoning. Place in oven and bake for about 20 minutes, or until thermometer reads at least 165 degrees. Serve warm.

Pecan Crusted Chicken 🍴 *(4 servings)*

½ cup mayonnaise
¼ cup Dijon mustard
2 tbsp. honey
4 (5 oz.) boneless chicken breasts
1 ½ cups finely chopped pecans

1 ½ cups gluten-free panko breadcrumbs
2 tsp. salt
1 ½ tsp. garlic powder
1 teaspoon paprika
½ tsp. black pepper

Preheat oven to 425 degrees. In a large bowl, combine mayonnaise, mustard, and honey, whisk together well. Add chicken and let marinate for a minimum of 30 minutes, or overnight. In a shallow bowl, toss together pecans, breadcrumbs, salt, garlic powder, paprika, and black pepper. Remove chicken pieces from marinade, add to pecan mixture and press down. Turn over and repeat so all sides are completely covered. Transfer chicken pieces to a greased 9x13 inch baking dish and add any remaining pecan mixture to top of chicken and press down evenly. Spray lightly with cooking spray. Bake chicken in oven until cooked through, about 25-30 minutes or until internal temperature reaches 165 degrees. Serve warm.

Poppyseed Chicken 🍴 *(4 servings)*

3 cups cooked chicken, diced
1 can gluten-free cream of chicken soup
8 oz. sour cream

1 tbsp. poppyseeds
1 ½ cups gluten-free panko breadcrumbs
¼ cup butter, melted

Preheat oven to 350 degrees. Combine chicken, soup, sour cream, and poppyseeds in a medium size mixing bowl and stir together. Spoon into a greased 11x7 inch baking dish. Combine breadcrumbs and melted butter in a small mixing bowl and toss together, sprinkle on top of chicken mixture. Bake for 30 minutes, serve warm.

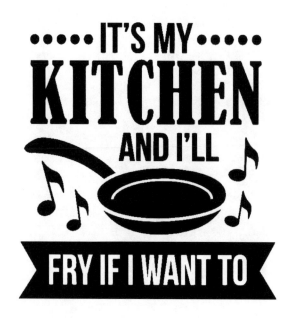

Quesadilla Lasagna *(6-8 servings)*

24 oz. sour cream
¼ cup jalapeno juice*
2 tbsp. granulated sugar
2 tbsp. cumin
2 tbsp. paprika
½ tbsp. garlic powder

½ tsp. ground cayenne
1 lb. cooked chicken, diced
2 cups grated pepper jack cheese
2 cups grated sharp cheddar cheese
18 corn tortillas
2 cups grated mozzarella cheese

Preheat oven to 350 degrees. In a large mixing bowl, combine the sour cream, garlic powder, cayenne, sugar, cumin, paprika, and jalapeno juice. Whisk together well. Stir in chicken, followed by pepper jack and sharp cheddar cheeses. Layer tortillas in greased 9x13 inch baking dish, spread a layer of chicken mixture on top. Repeat process two more times, then sprinkle mozzarella cheese on top. Bake in oven for 35-45 minutes, or until hot.

Pro-Tip: jalapeno juice is an important ingredient for superb flavor! Grab a can of jalapenos at the grocery store and use the juice, reserving the jalapenos for later.

Roasted Turkey Breast *(6-8 servings)*

¼ cup butter, softened
1 garlic clove, minced
1 tsp. paprika
1 tsp. Italian seasoning
½ tsp. onion powder
Salt and black pepper to taste

3 lb. turkey breast with skin
1 tbsp. butter
1 oz. dry white wine
1 cup chicken stock
3 tbsp. gluten-free all-purpose flour (no XG)
2 tbsp. heavy cream

Preheat oven to 350 degrees. In a small bowl, combine ¼ cup butter, garlic, paprika, Italian seasoning and onion powder, mix together well. Place turkey breast with skin side up in a roasting pan. Loosen skin with fingers, brush half of butter mixture over breast and under skin. Set aside remaining butter mixture. Sprinkle with salt and pepper, then loosely cover with aluminum foil. Place pan in oven and roast for 1 hour, remove from oven and brush with remaining butter mixture. Return to oven and roast for about 30 more minutes, or until an instant-read thermometer inserted into the thickest part reads 165 degrees. Remove from oven, let turkey rest for 10 minutes before serving. While turkey is resting, transfer pan drippings to a skillet and skim off excess grease. Cook over low heat, melt 1 tbsp. butter in skillet and add white wine. Scrape browned bits of food from skillet, then whisk in flour and cook for 1 minute. Slowly add chicken stock and whisk to prevent clumps from forming. Bring to a simmer, whisking constantly until thickened. Add heavy cream and stir, remove from heat. Slice turkey breast and serve with gravy.

Salsa Chicken (6-8 servings)

1 ½ lbs. cooked chicken, diced
15 oz. can black beans, drained
12 oz. bag frozen corn, thawed
1 tbsp. taco seasoning

2 (15.5 oz.) jars salsa
2 cups grated Mexican blend cheese
Mexican Rice (p. 190)

Preheat oven to 350 degrees. In a large mixing bowl, combine chicken, black beans, corn, taco seasoning, and salsa. Stir together very well. Spread into a greased 9x13 inch baking dish and sprinkle with grated cheese. Bake in oven for 35-45 minutes, or until hot and cheese is melted. Serve with Mexican Rice (p. 190).

Skillet Caprese Chicken (4 servings)

4 (5 oz.) boneless chicken breasts
½ tsp. garlic powder
½ tsp. onion powder
½ tsp. Italian seasoning
½ tsp. salt
¼ tsp. black pepper

2 tbsp. olive oil
6 oz. fresh mozzarella balls
2 medium tomatoes, sliced
Balsamic glaze
1/3 freshly chopped basil

Cover each piece of chicken with a piece of plastic wrap and pound with a meat mallet until even thickness, about ½ inch. Combine garlic powder, onion powder, Italian seasoning, salt and pepper in a small dish, stir to combine before sprinkling on both sides of each piece of chicken. Heat olive oil in a large skillet on medium heat. Add chicken and cook until golden brown on bottom, about 5-6 minutes. Turn chicken over and reduce heat to medium/low, cook for another 4-5 minutes. While chicken is cooking, slice mozzarella into 8 slices. Place 2 slices on each piece of chicken, followed by 2 slices of tomato on top of each piece of chicken. Cover pan and cook for 1-2 minutes, until cheese is melted, and chicken has reached an internal temperature of 165 degrees. Remove chicken from skillet, drizzle with balsamic glaze, sprinkle with fresh basil and serve warm.

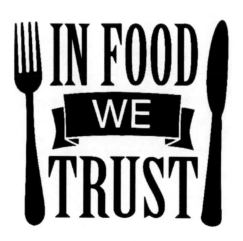

Slow Cooker Bacon Mushroom Chicken 🍴 *(6 servings)*

6 (5 oz.) boneless chicken breasts
½ cup real bacon bits
4 oz. can sliced mushrooms, drained

10 oz. can gluten-free cream of chicken soup
6 slices Swiss cheese

Spray a 6-quart slow cooker with cooking spray. Place chicken breasts in an even layer in slow cooker, sprinkle bacon bits on top. Drain mushrooms before layering on top of chicken, then spread chicken soup on top. Cover and cook on low for 4-5 hours, until meat thermometer reads 165 degrees. Place a slice of cheese on top of each piece of chicken, cover and cook for another 10 minutes or until cheese is melted. Serve warm.

Slow Cooker Roasted Chicken 🍴 *(6-8 servings)*

1 tbsp. paprika
2 tsp. salt
1 tsp. pepper

1 tsp. garlic powder
1 (4-5 lb.) whole chicken, giblets removed
1 whole onion, cut into thick pieces

In a small bowl, stir together paprika, salt, and garlic powder. Remove chicken from package, rub seasonings all over chicken, top and bottom. Place chopped onion into slow cooker to cover the bottom, lay chicken on top of onions, breast side up. Cook on low for 6-8 hours, or until a meat thermometer inserted in thickest part of chicken reaches internal temperature of at least 165 degrees. Cut chicken into pieces and serve.

What's the deal with the onion? The onion not only adds amazing flavor to the chicken, but also provides elevation for the chicken during the cooking process, which is key to cooking your chicken to perfection!

🍴 **Pro-Tip:** you can also buy a whole chicken that is already cut up for an easier way to serve. This way, you don't have to worry about cutting up the chicken, you just reach in there and grab some pieces...just don't use your hands. You know, food can get a little hot during the cooking process.

Slow Cooker Sesame Orange Chicken ▮ *(4-6 servings)*

2 tbsp. olive oil
2 lbs. boneless chicken breasts
1/3 cup cornstarch
½ tsp. salt
½ tsp. pepper
1 cup orange marmalade
¼ cup gluten-free soy sauce

1 tbsp. rice wine vinegar
1 tsp. sesame oil
½ tsp. ground ginger
½ tsp. garlic powder
2 tbsp. sesame seeds
2 tbsp. sliced green onions

Drizzle olive oil in bottom of a 4–6-quart slow cooker. Cut chicken breasts into 1-inch pieces, then place chicken in a large freezer bag, add cornstarch, salt, pepper, seal bag and toss to coat chicken evenly. Spread chicken into bottom of slow cooker. In a medium size mixing bowl, combine orange marmalade, soy sauce, rice wine vinegar, sesame oil, ginger, garlic powder, and whisk together to combine before pouring over chicken in slow cooker. Cover and cook on high for 2 hours or on low for 4 hours or until internal temperature of chicken is cooked through and no longer pink. Spoon chicken onto plate, garnish with sesame seeds and green onions, and serve with as much sauce as desired, along with rice and vegetables.

Slow Cooker Turkey Tenderloin ▮ *(6-8 servings)*

24 oz. package turkey tenderloins
¼ cup olive oil

2 tbsp. coconut aminos
1 tbsp. Montreal steak seasoning

Pour olive oil and coconut aminos into a slow cooker, then sprinkle seasoning evenly on bottom. Place both turkey tenderloins in pot, move around to coat bottom well before turning over and repeating process so that tenderloins are covered on both sides. Turn setting to low and cook for 2-3 hours, or until a thermometer reads at least 165 degrees. Turn setting to warm, cut into slices and serve.

▮ Pro-Tip: serve this with some Creamy Mashed Potatoes (p. 187) for pure bliss.

Southwest Turkey Legs ▮ *(4 servings)*

4 medium turkey drumsticks
¼ cup butter, melted

1 ½ tbsp. taco seasoning
cooking spray

Preheat oven to 450 degrees. Spray a roasting rack inside a rimmed roasting pan with cooking spray. Pat the turkey legs dry with paper towels, brush melted butter all over before rubbing them with seasoning. Place on roasting rack and spray each leg with a little more cooking spray. Roast, uncovered, for about 20 minutes or until skin is browned. Cover loosely with aluminum foil, continue roasting for about 30 more minutes or until a meat thermometer reads 165 degrees. Remove pan from oven and allow turkey legs to rest for 10 minutes before serving.

Spicy Fried Chicken Tenders *(6-8 servings)*

2 lbs. chicken breast tenderloins
2 tsp. salt, divided
1 tsp. pepper, divided
2 cups gluten-free all-purpose flour
1 cup buttermilk
1 tbsp. hot sauce

2 cups vegetable oil, for frying
1/3 cup butter
2 tsp. paprika
1 tsp. ground cayenne
½ tsp. garlic powder

Season both sides of chicken tenders with 1 tsp. salt and ½ tsp. pepper. Combine remaining salt and pepper with flour in a shallow bowl and whisk together. In another shallow bowl, combine buttermilk and pepper sauce, beat with a whisk. Dredge chicken tenders in flour, then buttermilk, and back in the flour mixture to coat completely. Heat oil in a skillet on medium high heat or 350 degrees. Fry half of the tenders in hot oil for 2-3 minutes on one side before turning over and cooking for another 2-3 minutes, until chicken is no longer pink in center or 165 degrees. Place on paper towels to drain while frying the remaining chicken tenders. In a small saucepan, melt butter on medium/low heat. Add paprika, cayenne, and garlic powder, whisk together until melted. Brush butter mixture over chicken tenders before serving.

Taco Chicken Mac 'n Cheese *(6-8 servings)*

½ cup butter
½ cup gluten-free all-purpose flour (no XG)
3 tbsp. taco seasoning
4 ½ cups whole milk

1 lb. gluten-free elbow pasta
1 lb. grated pepper jack cheese
1 ½ lbs. grated sharp cheddar cheese
1 lb. Fajita-style cooked chicken, diced

Preheat oven to 350 degrees. Melt butter in a pot on medium heat, whisk in flour and cook for 1 minute. Add taco seasoning and whisk together again. Slowly pour in milk, whisking to break up clumps of flour. Continue to cook on medium heat for about 10 minutes, whisking occasionally to make sure clumps don't form in the sauce. Cook pasta according to package directions for al dente, drain and set aside. When sauce has thickened, turn off heat and add pepper jack and 1 lb. cheddar, stirring until they have melted. Add chicken and pasta, stir well. Spoon into greased 9x13 inch baking dish, top with remaining grated cheddar. Bake in oven for 35-45 minutes, or until hot.

Taco Turkey Stuffed Peppers 🍴 *(8 servings)*

8 bell peppers (any colors)
1 tbsp. olive oil
1 onion, diced
½ tsp. salt
½ tsp. black pepper
1 tsp. ground cumin
1 tsp. dried oregano

1 tsp. paprika
3 cloves garlic, minced
1 lb. ground turkey
15 oz. can black beans, drained
15 oz. can corn, drained
16 oz. jar salsa
Guacamole, for serving

Preheat oven to 400 degrees. Cut off the tops of each bell pepper, cut out and remove seeds and ribs from the inside. Place each pepper on a lightly greased roasting pan and set aside. Heat olive oil in a large skillet on medium heat, add onion, salt, pepper, cumin, oregano, and paprika. Stir together well, cook until onion is tender. Add garlic and sauté until fragrant, about 30 seconds. Spread the onions and garlic to the sides of the pan to make room for the ground turkey. Cook turkey, breaking up and mixing with onions, until fully cooked. Add black beans, corn, and salsa, stir together well. Spoon mixture into peppers, place pepper tops back on and transfer pan to oven to roast for 30-35 minutes or until the peppers have softened and slightly wilted. Remove pan from oven, remove pepper tops and spoon guacamole on top of mixture. Replace pepper tops and serve warm.

Pro-Tip: green bell peppers have a more bitter taste, orange and yellow are slightly sweeter, and red bell peppers are the sweetest. For any stuffed bell pepper recipe, you can decide which peppers you would like to use, and even have a variety.

Thai Coconut Chicken 🍴 *(4 servings)*

1 cup full-fat coconut milk
1/3 cup creamy peanut butter
1 tbsp. coconut aminos
1 tbsp. lime juice
1 tbsp. brown sugar
¼ tsp. ground coriander

¼ tsp. ground cumin
1 tsp. ground ginger
2 tbsp. coconut oil
2 lbs. boneless chicken thighs
Salt and pepper, to taste

Combine coconut milk, peanut butter, coconut aminos, lime juice, brown sugar, coriander, cumin, and ginger in a medium size mixing bowl and whisk together well. Heat coconut oil in a large skillet on medium heat. Cut up chicken into bite-size pieces and season with salt and pepper before adding to skillet. Sauté chicken until cooked through, about 5-6 minutes. Give the sauce a quick whisk and add to pan with chicken. Once sauce is heated through, serve with rice and vegetables.

Toasted Almond Chicken *(6 servings)*

6 (5 oz.) boneless chicken breasts
Salt and pepper, to taste
¼ cup butter, divided
1 ½ cups heavy cream

2 tbsp. orange marmalade
1 tbsp. Dijon mustard
¼ tsp. paprika
2.25 oz. package sliced almonds

Place chicken between two pieces of heavy-duty plastic wrap and pound with a meat mallet to ¼ inch thick, sprinkle with salt and pepper. Melt 2 tbsp. butter in a skillet on medium/high heat, add 3 pieces of chicken and cook for 2-3 minutes on each side until golden. Remove chicken from skillet to a plate, repeat cooking with remaining butter and chicken. Reduce heat to medium, add heavy cream, orange marmalade, mustard, and paprika, stir well. Add chicken, sprinkle with almonds and continue cooking for another 8 minutes until sauce thickens. Serve warm.

Turkey Burgers *(4 servings)*

1 lb. ground turkey (80-90% lean)
½ cup diced red onion
¼ cup gluten-free panko breadcrumbs
½ tsp. garlic powder
1 egg, beaten

1 tsp. sea salt
1 tsp. onion powder
1 tsp. liquid smoke
½ tsp. dried Italian seasoning
¼ tsp. black pepper

Line a baking sheet with parchment paper and set aside. Combine all ingredients in a large mixing bowl and mix together well using clean hands. Divide the mixture into four equal portions and form them into patties. Place each patty on the lined baking sheet. Press a divot into the middle of each patty using your thumb (this will prevent the patties from shrinking during the cooking process on the grill). Place patties in refrigerator to chill for at least 30 minutes. Preheat grill to medium/high heat, around 450 degrees. Clean the grill well and grease. When the grill is heated, place patties on grill and cover, cook for 4-5 minutes. Gently turn patties over and cook for another 4-5 minutes, until internal temperature is 165 degrees. When burgers are ready, transfer to a clean plate and serve with gluten-free buns and toppings.

One of my favorite ways to eat a burger is wrapped in lettuce. If you would like to do the same, use larger pieces of lettuce to replace the top and bottom parts that a bun covers...just be prepared that it's a little bit messier than eating with a traditional bun. If you have mastered eating a lettuce-wrapped burger without making a mess, please teach me your method because I need a bib every time I do this. It's still worth it.

Turkey Meatballs 🍴 *(6-8 servings)*

2 lbs. ground turkey (93% lean)
1 cup gluten-free breadcrumbs
2/3 cup minced onion
½ cup minced fresh parsley
2 large eggs, beaten
3 cloves garlic, minced

2 tsp. gluten-free Worcestershire sauce
½ tsp. dried basil
½ tsp. dried oregano
1 tsp. sea salt
½ tsp. pepper
¼ cup olive oil

Preheat oven to 400 degrees. Combine all ingredients except olive oil in a large mixing bowl. Using clean hands, mix well until all ingredients are combined. Shape into 1-inch balls. Line a rimmed baking sheet with foil, coat a wire rack with cooking spray and set on top of baking sheet. Arrange meatballs on wire rack, brush with olive oil, and bake for 15-20 minutes or until internal thermometer reads 165 degrees. Serve warm.

🍴 **Pro-Tip:** to save extras for later, lay meatballs about 1 inch apart on a baking sheet lined with parchment paper and place in freezer. When meatballs are frozen, (about 1 hour), transfer to a zipper freezer bag, seal and store in freezer until ready to use. Reheat in microwave in small batches, 45-60 seconds or until hot. Serve warm.

Turkey Meatloaf 🍴 *(4-6 servings)*

For the Glaze
2/3 cup ketchup
1/3 cup light brown sugar

1 ½ tbsp. apple cider vinegar
1 tsp. Dijon mustard

For the Meatloaf
1 tbsp. olive oil
1 medium yellow onion, minced
3 cloves garlic, minced
1 tsp. sea salt
½ tsp. black pepper
2 tsp. paprika

1 tsp. dried thyme
1 ½ tbsp. gluten-free Worcestershire
1 ½ tsp. Dijon mustard
2 large eggs, beaten
2 lbs. ground turkey (93% lean)
¾ cup gluten-free seasoned breadcrumbs

Preheat oven to 350 degrees. In a small mixing bowl, combine all ingredients for glaze, whisk together and set aside. Heat olive oil in a small sauté pan over medium heat, add onion and cook until soft while stirring occasionally. Add the garlic and cook for 1 more minute, set aside to cool. In a large mixing bowl, combine all ingredients for meatloaf along with ¼ cup of glaze. Mix together well using clean hands. Transfer mixture to a meatloaf pan or shape into a loaf on a heavy-duty foil-lined rimmed baking sheet that has been greased with cooking spray. Spread remaining glaze mixture on top and place in oven to bake for 70-75 minutes, or until internal thermometer reads 165 degrees. Let rest for 5 minutes before serving.

Verde Chicken *(4 servings)*

16 oz. jar salsa verde
4 (5 oz.) boneless skinless chicken breasts
1 tbsp. olive oil
¼ tsp. sea salt
1/8 tsp. black pepper

1 tsp. garlic powder
2 cups grated Monterey jack cheese
3 Roma tomatoes, diced
1/3 cup chopped fresh cilantro

Preheat oven to 425 degrees. Grease a 9x13 inch baking dish with cooking spray and set aside. Place each piece of chicken between two pieces of plastic wrap and pound to 1 inch thickness. Lay chicken in baking dish, drizzle with olive oil and sprinkle with half of salt, pepper, and garlic powder. Turn chicken over and sprinkle remaining salt, pepper, and garlic powder. Pour the salsa verde on top of chicken into even layer, make sure all chicken is covered completely to keep it from drying out during the baking process. Top with grated cheese, place in oven to bake for 25 minutes or until internal temperature is 165 degrees. Remove dish from oven and sprinkle with diced tomatoes and cilantro. Serve with cauliflower rice, white rice or Mexican Rice (p. 190).

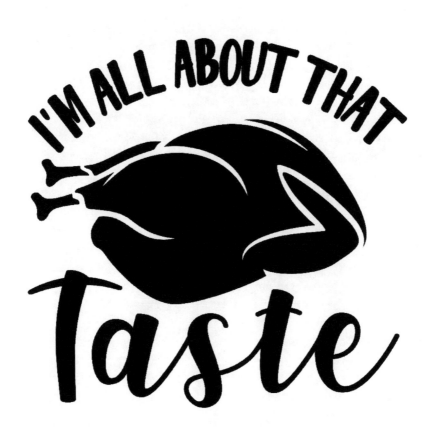

I'M ALL ABOUT THAT Taste

Beef, Pork & Seafood

Bacon Cheeseburger Casserole 🍴 *(4-6 servings)*

1 lb. ground hamburger
1 tbsp. hamburger seasoning
3 oz. package real bacon bits

16 oz. gluten-free frozen French fries
16 oz. sour cream
3 cups grated cheddar cheese, divided

Preheat oven to 400 degrees. In a medium skillet, cook hamburger on medium heat until browned and cooked completely. Coat 8x8 inch baking dish with cooking spray and evenly distribute French fries into dish. Drain meat and pour into a medium mixing bowl. Add hamburger seasoning and sour cream. Stir well. Add 2 cups grated cheddar and stir again. Spoon mixture on top of French fries into an even layer; sprinkle with remaining 1 cup cheddar and bacon bits. Place dish in oven. Bake for 30-35 minutes and serve warm.

🍴 **Pro-Tip:** mix it up for a variety! You can use different types of frozen French fries, just don't forget to adjust the baking time as needed. Hearty steak fries will take longer than those little skinny fries. We're also huge fans of tater tots, so you can easily turn this into a **Bacon Cheeseburger Tater Tot Casserole.** If that doesn't sound delicious, then I don't know what does.

Baked Ziti 🍴 *(6-8 servings)*

16 oz. uncooked gluten-free penne pasta
2 (24 oz.) jars spaghetti sauce
16 oz. ricotta cheese, at room temp

1 lb. ground beef
1 cup grated parmesan cheese
2 cups grated mozzarella cheese

In a skillet on high heat, cook ground beef until browned and drain excess liquid. Cook pasta according to package directions and drain. Preheat oven to 375 degrees. In a large mixing bowl, combine meat and ricotta cheese, beat with electric mixer. Add cooked pasta noodles and both jars of spaghetti sauce. Stir ingredients well and spoon into a 9x13 inch baking dish. Sprinkle Parmesan cheese evenly on top of pasta, followed by mozzarella cheese. Bake for 30 minutes, serve warm.

BBQ Bacon Burgers 🍴 *(6 servings)*

2 lbs. ground beef (80% lean)
½ cup gluten-free panko breadcrumbs
1 large egg, beaten

2 tbsp. BBQ seasoning
2 tbsp. milk
¼ cup real bacon bits

Combine all ingredients in a large mixing bowl and mix with hands until combined. Form into 6 equal size patties that are slightly larger than the buns and lay on a parchment paper lined baking sheet, then press down the center of each one with a spoon to keep them from puffing up while cooking. Preheat grill or skillet to medium heat (350-400 degrees), grill or fry for 3-4 minutes on each side. Serve warm on a gluten-free bun with your favorite toppings.

Beef and Broccoli ♟ *(4-6 servings)*

1 tsp. grated fresh ginger
3 cloves garlic, minced
½ cup hot water
6 tbsp. gluten-free soy sauce
3 tbsp. light brown sugar
1 ½ tbsp. cornstarch

¼ tsp. pepper
2 tbsp. sesame oil
1 lb. flank steak
2 tbsp. olive oil, divided
6 cups broccoli florets
2 tsp. sesame seeds

In a small mixing bowl, combine ginger, garlic, hot water, soy sauce, sugar, cornstarch, pepper, and sesame oil together. Whisk together and set aside. Slice flank steak into thin, bite-sized strips and set aside. Heat a large skillet on medium heat, add 1 tbsp. olive oil and broccoli florets, toss together. Cover and sauté for 4-5 minutes until broccoli is bright green and crisp/tender, then remove from pan. Add remaining 1 tbsp. olive oil and flank steak in a single layer, sauté for 2 minutes on each side or just until cooked through. Pull out a piece to test for doneness. Add sauce to skillet, reduce heat to medium/low and simmer for 3-4 minutes. Add broccoli and stir to combine, add 1-2 tbsp. water to thin sauce if desired. Serve warm with white rice.

Beefy Bean Enchiladas ♟ *(8 servings)*

1 lb. ground beef
15 oz. can refried beans
8 oz. sour cream
3 tbsp. taco seasoning

1 lb. grated sharp cheddar cheese
1 cup Fiesta blend grated cheese
16 corn tortillas
Enchilada Sauce (p. 86)

Preheat oven to 350 degrees. Heat a skillet on medium heat, cook ground beef until brown and fully cooked through. Drain and dump into a large mixing bowl. Add refried beans, sour cream, taco seasoning, and sharp cheddar cheese. Using an electric mixer, beat at medium speed until well combined. Scoop 1/3 cup of mixture into each tortilla. Spread into an even layer in the shape of a rectangle, about 1 inch from the sides of the tortilla. Tuck in the sides and roll up tortilla, place seam side down in greased 9x13 inch baking dish. Repeat process with remaining tortillas. Pour Enchilada Sauce (p. 86) on top and sprinkle with 1 cup Fiesta blend cheese. Bake in oven for 30 minutes, serve hot.

Pro-Tip: warm tortillas are much easier to work with when making enchiladas. Pop them on a microwave safe plate and heat for about 15-20 seconds, just until warmed and more pliable.

Beefy Rice Casserole *(6-8 servings)*

1 lb. ground beef
32 oz. beef broth
2 packets gluten-free French onion soup mix

1 cup long grain white rice
1 cup water

Preheat oven to 375 degrees. Cook ground beef in a skillet on medium heat until browned and fully cooked through, drain liquid from beef. In a large mixing bowl, whisk together beef broth and packets of soup mix. Add cooked beef, water, and rice. Stir together well, pour into 9x13 inch baking dish. Place dish in oven and bake for 45-50 minutes, until rice is tender. Serve warm.

Beef Stew *(6-8 servings)*

2 lbs. cubed beef stew meat
1 medium white onion
1.5 lbs. small red potatoes
3 medium carrots

32 oz. beef broth
1 packet gluten-free French onion soup mix
½ cup gluten-free all-purpose flour (no XG)

Cut onion into 1-inch pieces, red potatoes into quarters, and carrots into ½ inch circles. In a 4-quart slow cooker, add meat, onion, potatoes, and carrots. In a medium mixing bowl, whisk together the beef broth, flour, and onion soup mix. Pour into slow cooker, cook on low for 10-12 hours or high for 4-6 hours. Serve warm.

Pro-Tip: for a thicker stew, whisk together 2 tablespoons cornstarch with 2 tablespoons cold water. Pour into slow cooker about 30 minutes before serving, stir well. Stir again just before serving.

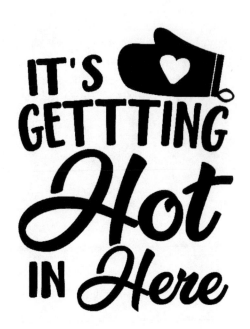

Beef Stroganoff ♨ *(4-6 servings)*

1 lb. ground beef
2 tbsp. butter
½ onion, diced
8 oz. brown mushrooms, sliced
1 garlic clove, minced
2 tbsp. gluten-free all-purpose flour (no XG)

1 cup beef broth
1 cup heavy cream
1 tbsp. gluten-free Worcestershire sauce
½ tsp. salt
¼ tsp. black pepper
8 oz. gluten-free pasta (elbow or penne)

Cook beef in a skillet on medium heat until browned and fully cooked through. Drain and set aside in a bowl. Add butter to skillet, when melted add onion and mushrooms. Cook until tender, about 6-8 minutes. Add garlic and sauté until fragrant, about 1 minute. Add flour and sauté for another minute, stirring constantly. Next, add beef broth and scrape any bits from the bottom before adding heavy cream and cooking for another 2 minutes or until slightly thickened. Add Worcestershire sauce, salt and pepper, stir together well. Cook pasta according to package directions, drain and add to beef mixture. Serve warm.

Beef Tenderloin ♨ *(8-10 servings)*

4-5 lb. beef tenderloin
1 tsp. salt
½ tsp. black pepper
2 tbsp. olive oil

¼ cup butter, softened
1 clove garlic, minced
1 tsp. Dijon mustard
1 tsp. dried thyme

Trim the beef tenderloin, then cut in half to make two pieces. Use butcher's twine to tie the tenderloin (see Pro Tip below). Rub salt and pepper all over and leave in refrigerator (uncovered) for at least 10 hours or overnight (this gives it a great crust, but not mandatory). Remove tenderloin from fridge 2 hours prior to cooking to allow it to come to room temperature. Preheat oven to 425 degrees. Heat oil in a large skillet on medium/high heat. Sear the tenderloin on all sides, about 3-5 minutes per side to create a nice golden crust and set aside. In a small bowl, combine butter, garlic, mustard, and dried thyme and mix before rubbing all over tenderloin and place in a baking dish or roasting pan. Place in preheated oven and roast until desired internal temperature, remove from oven and transfer to a cutting board. Let rest for 15-20 minutes before slicing into 1-inch pieces and serve with a big fat smile on your face.

RARE: 115-120 degrees F
MEDIUM RARE: 120-125 degrees F
MEDIUM: 130-135 degrees F

Pro-Tip: to save some time, you can ask your butcher to trim and tie the tenderloin for you, so it's ready to go. If you prefer to do it yourself but are a little rusty, check out YouTube for some how-to videos of how to tie a beef tenderloin. Beef Tenderloin is typically cooked rare-medium for best quality.

Beef Tips 🍴 *(4-6 servings)*

2 tbsp. olive oil
2 lbs. cubed chuck or stew meat
Salt and pepper, to taste
1 onion, diced
24 oz. beef broth

1 packet gluten-free French onion soup mix
1 tbsp. gluten-free Worcestershire sauce
¼ cup cornstarch
1/3 cup water

Heat 1 tbsp. Dutch oven or large pot on medium/high heat. Season meat with desired amount of salt and pepper, cook meat in small batches until browned, removed from pot and set aside. Reduce heat to medium, add remaining olive oil and onion. Cook until onion is soft, about 6-8 minutes. Add meat, beef broth, soup mix, and Worcestershire sauce to pot. Bring to a boil, cover and reduce heat to low to simmer for 1 1/2 -2 hours or until beef is fork tender. Combine cornstarch and water, whisk together well and pour slowly into beef mixture while stirring to thicken sauce to desired consistency. Taste and season with more salt and pepper, if desired. Serve warm with rice or mashed potatoes.

Carne Asada 🍴 *(6-8 servings)*

2 limes, juiced
4 cloves garlic, minced
½ cup orange juice
1 cup chopped fresh cilantro
½ tsp. salt

½ tsp. pepper
¼ olive oil
1 jalapeno, seeded and minced
2 tbsp. white vinegar
2 lbs. flank steak

In a small mixing bowl, combine lime juice, garlic, orange juice, cilantro, salt, pepper, olive oil, jalapeno, and vinegar, whisk to combine. Pour into a gallon size freezer bag and add flank steak. Seal up the bag tightly, massage to make sure the entire piece of meat is covered with marinade. Place in refrigerator for at least 2 hours, preferably overnight. When ready to cook, preheat grill to high heat (about 500 degrees). Remove steak from bag and discard marinade. Cook steak on the grill for about 8-10 minutes per side, or until done. Let meat rest for 10 minutes before slicing against the grain, serve warm with tacos or fajitas.

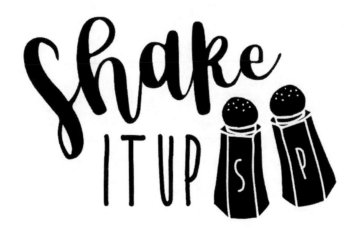

Cheese Tortellini *(8-10 servings)*

1 ½ lbs. ground beef
2 (28 oz.) cans crushed tomatoes
2 cups heavy cream
2 tbsp. granulated sugar
2 tbsp. onion powder
2 tbsp. garlic powder
2 tsp. dried oregano
2 tsp. dried basil
1 tsp. kosher salt
1 tsp. black pepper
3 lbs. gluten-free cheese tortellini
1 cup grated parmesan cheese
1 lb. grated mozzarella cheese

Preheat oven to 350 degrees. In a large pot on medium heat, cook ground beef until browned and drain excess liquid, return meat to pot. Add crushed tomatoes, heavy cream, and all dry seasonings to pot with meat and stir well. Continue to cook on medium heat for about 10 minutes. While sauce is cooking, cook pasta according to package directions for al dente, drain and set aside. When sauce is hot, add parmesan. Stir together well and continue cooking until cheese has melted. Remove pot from heat, add drained pasta and stir together well. Spoon into a greased 9x13 inch baking dish and bake in oven for 35-45 minutes, or until hot.

Cheeseburger Macaroni *(8-10 servings)*

1 lb. ground beef
½ cup butter
½ cup gluten-free all-purpose flour (no XG)
4 cups whole milk
1 tbsp. Dijon mustard
½ tbsp. kosher salt
1 tbsp. paprika
½ tsp. black pepper
½ tsp. garlic powder
½ tsp. onion powder
¼ teaspoon cayenne pepper (optional)
2 lbs. grated sharp cheddar cheese, divided
2 lbs. gluten-free elbow pasta

Preheat oven to 350 degrees. In a large skillet on medium heat, cook ground beef until browned and drain excess liquid, set aside. Melt butter in a pot at medium heat, whisk in flour and cook for 1 minute. Add seasonings and whisk together again. Slowly pour in milk, whisking to break up clumps of flour. Continue to cook on medium heat for about 10 minutes, whisking occasionally to make sure clumps don't form in the sauce. Cook pasta according to package directions for al dente, drain and set aside. When sauce has thickened, turn off heat and add 1 ½ lbs. cheddar cheese, stirring until it has melted. Add cooked hamburger and pasta, stir well. Spread into a greased 9x13 inch baking dish and sprinkle with remaining cheddar. Bake in oven for 35-45 minutes, or until hot.

Chili Cornbread Casserole *(6-8 servings)*

For the Chili
2 lbs. ground beef
1 tbsp. chili powder
1 tsp. onion powder
1 tsp. cumin
1 tsp. garlic powder
28 oz. can crushed tomatoes
15 oz. can black beans, drained
Salt and pepper, to taste

For the Cornbread Topping
1 cup gluten-free cornmeal
1 cup gluten-free all-purpose flour
1 tsp. salt
1 tbsp. granulated sugar
2 tsp. baking powder
1 cup milk
2 eggs
6 tbsp. butter, melted

Preheat oven to 375 degrees. Grease an 8x8 inch baking dish or 9-inch deep dish pie plate with cooking spray and set aside. Heat skillet on medium heat and cook ground beef until browned and fully cooked through. Remove from heat and drain meat. Return cooked meat to skillet, add chili powder, onion powder, cumin, garlic powder, and stir together. Stir in crushed tomatoes and black beans, season with salt and pepper to taste. Simmer for another 5-7 minutes, then spoon into casserole dish. In a large mixing bowl, whisk together cornmeal, flour, salt, sugar, and baking powder. In a small mixing bowl, combine milk, eggs, and melted butter, whisk together well and pour into bowl with dry ingredients. Stir together until well combined, then spread into an even layer on top of chili mixture in casserole dish. Bake for 30-35 minutes or until cornbread is lightly golden. Serve warm.

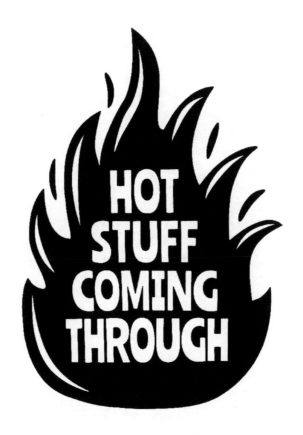

Chipotle Ribeye Steaks (4 servings)

3 cloves garlic, minced
7 oz. can chipotle peppers in adobo sauce
2 tbsp. olive oil
2 tsp. cumin

2 tsp. dried oregano
1 tbsp. salt
½ tsp. pepper
4 ribeye steaks

In a food processor, combine garlic, chipotle peppers (with sauce), olive oil, cumin, dried oregano, salt, and pepper. Process until smooth, add water as needed. In large zipper freezer bags, combine steaks and marinade. You will need multiple bags, so be sure to distribute the marinade evenly. Seal bags and massage steaks to make sure they are completely coated with marinade. Set aside and marinate for 1 hour at room temperature or up to 12 hours in refrigerator. **Make sure your steaks are at room temperature before cooking.** Preheat your grill, remove steaks from marinade bags and place on grill to cover and cook for 4-5 minutes per side or until desired temperature. Remove steaks from grill and let rest for about 10 minutes before serving.

RARE: 125-130 degrees
MEDIUM RARE: 130-140 degrees
MEDIUM: 140-150 degrees

MEDIUM WELL: 150-160 degrees
WELL: Over 160 degrees

Country Fried Steak (4 servings)

4 (8 oz. each) cube steaks
½ tbsp. salt
1 tsp. black pepper
2 large eggs
2 ¾ cups whole milk, divided
1 ½ cups gluten-free all-purpose flour
1 tsp. garlic powder

1 tsp. onion powder
1 tsp. paprika
1 cup vegetable oil
3 tbsp. butter
3 tbsp. gluten-free all-purpose flour (no XG)
½ cup heavy cream

Preheat oven to 225 degrees. Place one piece of steak on a cutting board, cover with plastic wrap and pound the steak evenly to ¼ inch thick using a meat mallet, season with salt and pepper on both sides. In a wide, shallow dish, combine eggs and 1 cup milk, whisk together well and set aside. In another shallow dish, combine 1 ½ cups flour, garlic powder, onion powder, and paprika, whisk together well. Dredge steak in flour mixture, then dip into egg mixture. Return to flour mixture again and coat well, set aside while repeating process for each steak. Heat vegetable oil in a large skillet over medium heat. When oil is hot, fry the steaks two at a time for 3 minutes on each side until golden brown and internal temperature reaches 155-165 degrees. Transfer steaks to a baking sheet lined with paper towels. When all steaks are finished frying, transfer to oven to keep warm while preparing the gravy. Discard hot oil from frying pan but leave any browned bits. Melt butter on medium heat, add 3 tbsp. flour and whisk to incorporate. Cook for 2-3 minutes, add heavy cream and remaining milk. Bring to a simmer and cook, whisking constantly for 5-7 minutes or until thickened. Season with salt and pepper, smother steaks with gravy when ready to serve.

Hamburger Steak ⚔ (4 servings)

1 lb. ground beef
¼ cup gluten-free breadcrumbs
1 egg, beaten
1 tsp. gluten-free Worcestershire sauce
1 tbsp. Montreal steak seasoning

1 tbsp. vegetable oil
2 tbsp. gluten-free all-purpose flour (no XG)
1 cup beef broth
1 packet gluten-free French onion soup mix

Combine ground beef, breadcrumbs, egg, Worcestershire, and steak seasoning in a medium size mixing bowl and mix well with hands. Form into 8 equal size patties and set aside. Heat oil in skillet on medium heat and fry patties until nicely browned, about 4 minutes per side. Transfer cooked patties to a plate. Add flour to pan and whisk, scraping bits of beef off the bottom. Slowly pour in beef broth while whisking, then add onion soup mix and whisk again. Simmer and stir until gravy thickens, about 5 minutes. Reduce heat to low, return patties to pan with gravy, cover and simmer until cooked through, about 10-15 minutes. Serve warm.

Lasagna ⚔ (10-12 servings)

2 lbs. ground beef
2 (28 oz.) cans crushed tomatoes
8 oz. can tomato sauce
½ cup grated parmesan cheese
32 oz. ricotta cheese, room temp
2 eggs, beaten
2 tbsp. granulated sugar
2 tbsp. onion powder

2 tbsp. garlic powder
2 tsp. dried oregano
2 tsp. dried basil
1 tsp. kosher salt
1 tsp. black pepper
1 lb. gluten-free lasagna noodles
2 lbs. grated mozzarella cheese

Preheat oven to 350 degrees. In a large pot on medium heat, cook ground beef until browned and drain excess liquid, return meat to pot. Add crushed tomatoes, tomato sauce, and all dry seasonings to pot with meat and stir well. Continue to cook on medium heat for about 10 minutes, stirring occasionally. While sauce is cooking, cook pasta according to package directions for al dente, drain and set aside. Spoon a small amount of sauce in the bottom of a greased 9x13 inch baking dish. Lay one layer of lasagna noodles on top of sauce. In a mixing bowl, combine eggs, parmesan, and ricotta, beat with electric mixer until smooth. Spread half of ricotta mixture on top of noodles, followed by meat sauce and sprinkled with mozzarella. Repeat layers one more time. Bake in oven for 35-45 minutes, or until hot. Let sit for 5-10 minutes before serving.

London Broil 👥 *(6-8 servings)*

2 lbs. London Broil
2 cloves garlic, minced
¼ cup balsamic vinegar
¼ cup gluten-free Worcestershire sauce
2 tbsp. gluten-free soy sauce
2 tbsp. Dijon mustard

2 tbsp. olive oil
2 tbsp. light brown sugar
1 tsp. Italian seasoning
¼ tsp. salt
¼ tsp. black pepper
1 tbsp. vegetable oil

Place the steak on a cutting board and pound on both sides using the ridged side of a meat mallet. In a small mixing bowl, combine garlic, balsamic vinegar, Worcestershire, soy sauce, Dijon mustard, olive oil, brown sugar, Italian seasoning, salt and pepper, whisk together well. Pour marinade into large zipper plastic bag, add the steak and seal the bag. Massage the bag with your hands to make sure the meat is completely covered with the marinade. Refrigerate for 12-14 hours, turning over several times. Remove steak from bag, discard the marinade, and thoroughly dry steak with paper towels. Heat vegetable oil in a large skillet on medium/high heat. Add steak to pan and place a heavy bottom skillet on top of the meat to weigh it down while it sears. Cook for 6-7 minutes, then flip over and repeat process. Remove steak from pan and transfer to a cutting board to rest for 10 minutes before slicing into thin strips against the grain and serve warm.

Meatloaf 🥄 *(6-8 servings)*

For the Meatloaf
2 lbs. ground beef (80-85% lean)
1 egg, lightly beaten
1 tsp. garlic powder
1 tbsp. onion powder
1 tbsp. Worcestershire sauce
1 cup milk
1 cup gluten-free breadcrumbs
1/3 cup ketchup

For the Topping
1 tbsp. light brown sugar
1 tbsp. Dijon mustard
1/3 cup ketchup

Preheat oven to 350 degrees. Combine all ingredients for meatloaf in a large mixing bowl and mix well with hands. Place into a meatloaf pan, or shape into loaf and place in 9x13 inch baking dish. Combine ingredients for topping in a small bowl, stir together well, and spoon on top of meatloaf. Bake for 70-75 minutes, or until internal temperature reaches 155 degrees. Remove pan from oven; let meatloaf rest for 10 minutes before serving. Slice into 6-8 pieces and serve warm

Pro-Tip: meatloaf pans are AMAZING when it comes to making meatloaf. The geniuses who designed it made sure you can pull the whole loaf out of the pan without bringing all the fatty juices with it. Also makes it easier for slicing into cute little rectangles. Genius.

Mexican Casserole ⍾ *(6-8 servings)*

1 lb. ground beef
1 (1.25 oz.) packet taco seasoning
1 (20 oz.) can refried beans
16 oz. sour cream

1 (15 oz.) jar salsa
20 corn tortillas
4 cups grated Mexican blend cheese

Preheat oven to 375 degrees. Cook beef in skillet on medium heat until browned and fully cooked through, adding taco seasoning and stirring when beef is almost done. Remove from heat, stir in salsa and set aside. Coat a 9x13 inch baking dish with cooking spray. Layer 10 corn tortillas on bottom. In a medium size mixing bowl, combine refried beans and sour cream. Beat at medium speed with electric mixer until well blended. Spoon half of bean mixture on top of tortillas, spread into even layer. Spread half of beef and salsa mixture on top into even layer, then sprinkle 2 cups of cheese on top of beef. Repeat layering. Bake for 30 minutes, serve warm.

Pro-Tip: if getting your family to eat the contents of chunky salsa is an issue, just pour the salsa in a blender and puree until smooth. No chunks! You can also choose how hot or mild your dish is by how hot or mild the salsa is! Picante style salsa also has a smoother consistency.

Pan-Seared Steak ⍾ *(4 servings)*

2 lbs. New York Strip steaks
½ tbsp. vegetable oil
½ tbsp. salt

½ tsp. black pepper
2 tbsp. butter
2 cloves garlic, minced

Pat steaks dry using paper towels. Season each side with salt and pepper, let sit for about 30 minutes before cooking. When ready to cook, heat a cast iron pan on medium/high heat until hot, add vegetable oil and swirl to coat. Once the oil is very hot, add steaks to pan and sear on each side for 3-4 minutes until a brown crust has formed. Using tongs, turn the steak on its sides to sear the edges for 1 minute. Reduce heat to medium/low, add butter and garlic. Spoon sauce over steaks, continue cooking until steaks are 5-10 degrees from your desired doneness (temp will continue to rise while resting). Remove pan from heat, transfer steaks to a cutting board, loosely cover and let rest for 10 minutes before serving. Slice steaks into ½ inch strips and spoon extra butter sauce on top to serve.

RARE: 125-130 degrees F
MEDIUM RARE: 130-140 degrees F
MEDIUM: 140-150 degrees F

MEDIUM WELL: 150-160 degrees F
WELL: Over 160 degrees F

Pepper Steak 🍴 *(4-6 servings)*

1 tbsp. vegetable oil, divided
1 red bell pepper
1 green bell pepper
1 ¼ lbs. flank steak, thinly sliced
Salt and pepper to taste

2 cloves garlic, minced
1 tsp. minced ginger
¼ cup gluten-free soy sauce
2 tbsp. light brown sugar
2 tbsp. cornstarch

Heat 1 tsp. vegetable oil over medium heat in a large skillet pan. Core, seed, and cut each bell pepper into strips, place in pan to cook for 3-4 minutes or just until tender. Transfer peppers from pan to a plate. Add remaining 2 tsp. oil to pan, season steak with salt and pepper to taste. Increase heat to medium/high, add steak to pan and cook for 5-6 minutes on each side until lightly browned. Add garlic and ginger, cook for 30 seconds, then add peppers back to pan with steak. In a small bowl, combine soy sauce, sugar, cornstarch, and ¼ cup water, whisk together well. Pour sauce over steak mixture and continue cooking for 2-3 more minutes or until sauce has thickened. Serve warm.

Philly Cheesesteak Sandwiches 🍴 *(4 servings)*

4 gluten-free hoagie rolls
½ lb. thinly sliced deli roast beef
8 slices provolone cheese

2 green bell peppers, sliced
1 onion, sliced
1 tablespoon butter

Set oven to (high) broil. In a skillet on medium heat, melt butter. Add peppers and onions, stir occasionally while sautéing. Split hoagie rolls in half. Place on baking sheet with the split side up. On the bottom 4 pieces of rolls, evenly distribute roast beef on each one. Break each piece of cheese in half. Place 4 halves on the top 4 pieces of rolls. Place baking sheet in oven and broil for 2-4 minutes, until cheese is melted. Continue cooking vegetables until they are soft, while sandwiches are in oven. Remove baking sheet from oven and spoon cooked vegetables on top of roast beef. Place the top halves of rolls on top of the bottom. Serve warm.

Try not to run off and check social media while this is broiling in the oven. When the broil is set on high, it doesn't waste any time toasting your buns, and you don't want to come back to charred buns and sticky cheese. Yuck and ouch.

🍴 **Pro-Tip:** my favorite brand of gluten-free hoagie rolls to use is Udi® and they are typically found in the freezer section if your grocery store carries them. If you can't get your hands on hoagie rolls, hamburger buns will work too!

Prime Rib 🍴 *(4 servings)*

4 lb. bone-in beef prime rib
1 tbsp. salt, divided
½ tbsp. pepper
½ tsp. dried rosemary

¼ tsp. dried thyme
3 cloves garlic, minced
¼ cup butter, softened

Place prime rib on a plate and bring to room temperature, a minimum of 2-4 hours. ***This step is crucial for the cooking formula!!*** Preheat oven to 500 degrees. In a small bowl, combine ½ tsp. salt, pepper, rosemary, thyme, garlic, and butter, mix together well. Spread butter mixture evenly over entire roast and place on a rimmed baking sheet, then season generously with remaining salt. Multiply exact weight of roast by 5 minutes to determine your cooking time (4.2 x 5 = 21 minutes). Roast meat according to this calculation. When time is up, turn off oven and leave the roast in the oven with the door closed to rest for 2 hours. Step away from the oven for these 2 hours while it rests, don't even look at it. Remove from oven, slice bones off bottom and cut into 4 pieces and serve warm with au jus.

Shepherd's Pie 🍴 *(6-8 servings)*

2 lbs. ground beef
3 tbsp. tomato paste
¾ cup beef broth
½ tbsp. gluten-free Worcestershire sauce
½ tsp. dried thyme
1 tbsp. onion powder
1 tbsp. Montreal steak seasoning

1 bag frozen steam 'n mash potatoes*
1 cup whole milk
¾ cup unsalted butter
½ tsp. salt
¼ tsp. pepper
12 oz. bag frozen peas/carrots
2 cups grated sharp cheddar cheese

Preheat oven to 350 degrees. Cook ground beef in pot on medium heat until browned and cooked through. Drain meat, put back in pot. Add tomato paste, broth, Worcestershire, thyme, onion powder, and steak seasoning. Stir together well. Spoon into the bottom of your greased freezer containers into an even layer. Heat potatoes according to package directions, transfer to a mixing bowl and mash well. Heat milk and butter in a pot until hot and butter is melted, pour over potatoes, add salt and pepper, beat with electric mixer until smooth. Sprinkle peas and carrots on top of meat, spread mashed potatoes on top in an even layer and sprinkle with cheddar cheese. Bake for 35-45 minutes at 350 degrees.

Pro-Tip: not every grocery store carries these frozen steam 'n mash potatoes, but they are an amazing way to make quick and easy mashed potatoes.

Sloppy Joes (4 servings)

1 lb. ground beef (90% lean)
15 oz. can tomato sauce
1 tbsp. gluten-free Worcestershire sauce
½ tbsp. Dijon mustard
1 tbsp. light brown sugar

1 tsp. onion powder
1 tsp. garlic powder
½ tsp. salt
¼ tsp. pepper
4 gluten-free hamburger buns

Place a large skillet over medium heat and add ground beef. Sauté for about 5 minutes, or until cooked through and no longer pink, breaking it up with a spatula. In a small mixing bowl, combine tomato sauce, Worcestershire, mustard, brown sugar, onion powder, garlic powder, salt, and pepper, whisk together well. Drain beef, return to skillet and add sauce. Stir together well, reduce heat to low and cook for about 10 minutes until thickened and hot. For a thinner consistency, add water as needed. Toast hamburger buns if desired and serve as a regular or open-faced sandwich.

Steak Fajitas (6-8 servings)

2 lbs. flank steak
1 red bell pepper
1 green bell pepper
1 onion, sliced
3 tbsp. olive oil
1 tbsp. lime juice

1 tsp. chili powder
1 tsp. ground cumin
½ tsp. salt
½ tsp. black pepper
2 cloves garlic, minced
10-12 corn tortillas

Slice steak into ½ inch strips and place in a resealable freezer bag. Seed and slice bell peppers and place in another resealable freezer bag with onion. In a small bowl, combine olive oil, lime juice, chili powder, cumin, salt, pepper, and garlic, whisk together well. Pour 1/3 into bag with meat, 1/3 into bag with veggies, and reserve remaining 1/3 for when you're ready to cook. Seal bags tightly and refrigerate for at least one hour or up to overnight. When ready to cook, heat a large skillet over medium/high heat. Add vegetables to skillet and cook just until tender, about 5 minutes. Remove veggies from skillet and set aside on a plate. Add steak strips to skillet, cook for about 7-10 minutes. Add vegetables and reserved marinade to skillet, stir together and serve warm with tortillas. Garnish with sour cream, cheese, guacamole, salsa, shredded lettuce, Mexican Rice (p. 190), refried beans, etc.

Swedish Meatballs 🍴 *(4-6 servings)*

½ lb. ground beef
½ lb. ground pork
¼ gluten-free panko breadcrumbs
1 tsp. dried parsley
¼ tsp. ground allspice
¼ tsp. nutmeg
1 tsp. onion powder
½ tsp. garlic powder

½ tsp. salt
1 egg, beaten
6 tbsp. butter, divided
3 tbsp. gluten-free all-purpose flour (no XG)
2 cups beef broth
1 cup heavy cream
1 tbsp. gluten-free Worcestershire sauce
1 tsp. Dijon mustard

In a medium size mixing bowl, combine ground beef, pork, breadcrumbs, parsley, allspice, nutmeg, onion powder, garlic powder, salt, and egg. Mix with hands until combined, roll into 12 large meatballs or 20 small meatballs. Heat a large skillet on medium heat, add 2 tbsp. butter. When melted, add meatballs and cook, turning continuously until brown on each side and cooked through. Remove meatballs to make sauce. Add remaining butter and flour to skillet, whisk and cook until light brown. Slowly add beef broth and heavy cream, whisking to break up any clumps. Add Worcestershire and mustard, cook until it starts to thicken. Add salt and pepper to taste, if needed. Add meatballs back to skillet and cook for another 2-3 minutes. Serve over gluten-free noodles or rice.

Taco Spaghetti 🍴 *(4-6 servings)*

1 tbsp. olive oil
1 lb. ground beef
½ medium onion, diced
1 packet gluten-free taco seasoning
10 oz. can Rotel tomatoes

8 oz. gluten-free spaghetti noodles
3 cups water
1 cup grated sharp cheddar cheese
½ cup chopped fresh cilantro

Heat olive oil in a large skillet or Dutch oven over medium heat. Cook ground beef and onion until the meat is no longer pink and onion is soft. Add taco seasoning and Rotel tomatoes, stir together. Add water and spaghetti noodles, stir again. Bring to a boil, reduce heat to low, cover and cook for 13-15 minutes, until noodles are tender. Remove from heat, add cheese and stir. Garnish with fresh cilantro and serve warm.

Bacon Wrapped Pork Tenderloin 🍴 (4-6 servings)

8-10 pieces uncooked bacon
Pork tenderloin (approx. 1 ½ lbs.)

2 tablespoons maple syrup

Preheat oven to 375 degrees. Line a roasting pan with aluminum foil. Lay slices of bacon slighting overlapping each other on a cutting board. Unwrap tenderloin from package, place in the middle of the bacon slices. Slowly roll up the tenderloin with the bacon, secure with toothpicks. Place tenderloin on rack in roasting pan, place in oven. Cook for about 45-50 minutes, until meat thermometer inserted in center reads at least 145 degrees. Remove pan from oven, drizzle maple syrup over bacon, let rest for 5 minutes before cutting into slices and serving.

BBQ Garlic Pork Tenderloin 🍴 (4-6 servings)

1 pork tenderloin (about 1 ½ pounds)
1 cup gluten-free BBQ sauce
¼ cup light brown sugar

2 tbsp. Dijon mustard
1 clove garlic, minced

Place pork tenderloin in slow cooker. In a small mixing bowl, whisk together BBQ sauce, sugar, mustard, and garlic. Spoon sauce on top of pork tenderloin in slow cooker. Cook on low heat for 4 hours, or until thermometer measures at least 145 degrees. Remove tenderloin from slow cooker, slice into pieces, and drizzle sauce from pot over top. Serve warm.

BBQ Pork Fried Rice 🍴🍴 (6-8 servings)

¼ cup BBQ dry rub
1 lb. pork tenderloin
½ cup gluten-free BBQ sauce
2 tbsp. vegetable oil, divided
3 eggs, beaten
1 onion, diced
2 cloves garlic, minced

5 cups cooked rice (cold)
1 ½ cups frozen peas, thawed
2 tsp. toasted sesame oil
¼ cup gluten-free soy sauce
1 tbsp. grated fresh ginger
1 tsp. BBQ dry rub

Preheat oven to 375 degrees. Place pork on a baking sheet and cook in oven for 15 minutes. Remove from oven, cover the top with BBQ sauce and place back in the oven for another 8-10 minutes. While pork is cooking, heat 1 tbsp. vegetable oil in a large skillet or wok. Pour in beaten eggs, scramble, remove from pan and set aside. Add remaining vegetable oil and onion, cook until slightly tender, about 5 minutes. Add garlic and cook for another minute, until fragrant. Next add cooked rice to the pan, peas, eggs, soy sauce, sesame oil, grated ginger, and dry rub. Stir together to combine, turn heat to low and cook until heated through. When pork is done cooking and reaches an internal temperature of 145 degrees, slice into ½ inch pieces, then into cubes. Add pork to rice, stir to combine and serve warm.

Beanie Weenie® (4-6 servings)

1 lb. cooked sausage links   28 oz. can baked beans

Cut sausage into ½ inch thick coins and combine with beans in a pot on medium heat. Cook for 5-10 minutes, until hot and steaming. Serve warm to your favorite adults who still love to act like kids. No really, that's it...doesn't get much simpler than that.

If you're wondering why in the world this recipe is even in this book, it's because as a kid I absolutely LOVED eating Beanie Weenie® every time I went to my Granddad's house. One day I kinda grew up and wanted an adult version of this childhood favorite. Not only is it larger servings than the little individual serving cans, but also has a heartier meat by using sausage. These days, you can mix and match the type of baked beans with the type of sausage. For more of a kick, use spicy sausage along with a spicy blend of baked beans. Most baked beans that I have seen at the store these days are gluten-free, just make sure to triple check the ingredients.

Cajun Alfredo (6-8 servings)

1 cup butter   1 tsp. salt
¼ cup gluten-free all-purpose flour (no XG)   1 cup grated parmesan
3 tbsp. Cajun seasoning   12 oz. andouille sausage, sliced
1 quart half and half   12 oz. frozen cooked shrimp, thawed
1 cup heavy cream   1 lb. grated mozzarella cheese
1 lb. gluten-free penne pasta

Preheat oven to 350 degrees. Melt butter in pot on medium heat until melted, then whisk in flour and Cajun seasoning. Slowly add half and half and heavy cream, whisk and continue to cook for about 12-15 minutes, stirring occasionally. While the sauce is cooking, cook the pasta according to package directions in a separate pot just until al dente, drain and set aside. When sauce has thickened, reduce heat to low, stir in salt and grated parmesan. Remove pot from heat, stir in sausage, shrimp, and pasta. Spread into a greased 9x13 inch baking dish, sprinkle with mozzarella cheese. Bake in oven for 30-40 minutes, until hot and cheese is melted.

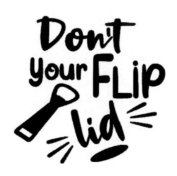

Cajun Mac 'n Cheese 🍴 *(6-8 servings)*

½ cup unsalted butter
1 cup gluten-free all-purpose flour (no XG)
4 ½ cups whole milk
2 tbsp. Cajun seasoning

1 tsp. kosher salt
1 lb. gluten-free elbow pasta
2 lbs. grated sharp cheddar cheese
1 lb. andouille sausage

Preheat oven to 350 degrees. Melt butter in a large pot on medium heat. When the butter is melted, whisk in the flour and cook for another minute. Slowly whisk in the milk, Cajun seasoning and salt. Continue to cook on medium heat, whisking occasionally to break up any clumps from the roux (butter and flour mixture). While the sauce is cooking, cook the pasta according to package directions until al dente; drain and set aside. When the sauce has been cooking for about 12-15 minutes and has thickened, reduce heat to low and stir in 1 ½ lbs. cheese using a large spoon (if you use the whisk, the cheese will clump up and get all caught up in it). Continue stirring until cheese has completely melted. Slice sausage into ½ inch coins and set aside. Remove pot from heat, stir in cooked pasta and sausage. Spread into a greased 9x13 inch baking dish and sprinkle with remaining cheese. Bake for 35-45 minutes, let sit for 5 minutes before serving.

Pro-Tip: this can also be pre-made and heated in a crock pot! Prepare as directed, then pour into a crock pot. I've made this 2-3 days in advance, stored it in the refrigerator and heated on low for 2-3 hours, stirring occasionally until hot and ready to eat. Great for potluck!

Carolina BBQ Ribs 🍴 *(4-6 servings)*

2-2 ½ lbs. baby back pork ribs
2 tbsp. BBQ rub

gluten-free BBQ sauce

Preheat oven to 275 degrees. Remove thin membrane covering the back of the rack of ribs. Season both sides with BBQ rub, place ribs meat side up into a large roasted pan or rimmed baking sheet. If you need to cut ribs in half to fit on pan, go for it. Cover the pan or baking sheet tightly with aluminum foil and bake for about 2 ½ - 3 ½ hours, until the meat falls off easily from the bones. Remove ribs from oven and brush generously on both sides with BBQ sauce, serve warm.

Pro-Tip: removing the membrane is what helps the meat fall off the bones when you take a bite. If you prefer a chewier consistency, leave the membrane on. You can also ask your butcher to remove the membrane for you to save a step for yourself at home.

Chinese BBQ Spareribs *(10-12 servings)*

½ cup gluten-free teriyaki sauce
¼ cup gluten-free soy sauce
3 tbsp. dark brown sugar
2 tbsp. honey

1 tbsp. five-spice powder
1 tsp. garlic powder
½ tsp. ground ginger
2 racks spareribs, sliced into singles

In a small mixing bowl, combine teriyaki sauce, soy sauce, sugar, honey, spice powder, garlic powder, and ground ginger, whisk together well. Reserve ¼ cup for later. Pour remaining sauce into a resealable freezer bag, add ribs and seal bag. Massage to make sure ribs are completely covered with sauce. Let marinate for at least 3 hours or preferably overnight. When ready to cook, preheat oven to 300 degrees. Place ribs meaty side up on a rimmed baking sheet and cover pan tightly with foil. Cook in oven for 1 hour 45 minutes. Remove foil and brush ribs with remaining sauce, increase oven temp to 350 degrees and bake uncovered for another hour. They should come out sticky and glazed, serve warm.

Corn Dogs *(6 servings)*

6 bamboo skewers or lollipop sticks
6 gluten-free hot dogs
½ cup gluten-free cornmeal
½ cup gluten-free all-purpose flour (no XG)
1 tbsp. granulated sugar

2 tsp. baking powder
½ tsp. salt
½ cup milk
1 egg, beaten
vegetable oil, for frying

Insert skewers or sticks into hot dogs, set aside. In a small mixing bowl, combine cornmeal, flour, sugar, baking powder, salt, milk, and egg. Whisk until very smooth, then transfer into a tall glass or mason jar and set in refrigerator to thicken. Pat hot dogs completely dry with paper towels (this will help the batter stick to the hot dog). Toss the hot dogs in extra flour until completely coated and set aside. Line a plate or platter with paper towels and heat at least 2-3 inches of oil in fryer or skillet pan on medium/high heat to 350 degrees. Remove batter from refrigerator and whisk again. Holding the stick of the hot dog, slowly dip each one into the batter and remove slowly to let it adhere to the hot dog. Allow excess batter to drip off, then dip it back in again. Twist it slowly after removing to help it stay on the hot dog. Gently place the hot dog in hot oil and fry for about 2 minutes on each side until golden and crispy all over. Remove from oil and set on paper towels to catch excess grease, serve warm with honey mustard or ketchup.

Crispy Sweet and Sour Pork 🍴 *(4-6 servings)*

For the Pork
1 lb. pork roast
½ onion, diced
1 clove garlic, minced
1 tsp. minced ginger
½ tsp. baking soda
2 tsp. cornstarch
2 tbsp. gluten-free soy sauce
¾ cup cornstarch, divided
Canola oil, for frying

For the Sauce
1/3 cup granulated sugar
1/3 cup apple cider vinegar
¼ cup pineapple juice
3 tbsp. ketchup
1 tsp. gluten-free Worcestershire sauce
1 tbsp. gluten-free soy sauce
1 tbsp. cornstarch
¼ cup water

Cut pork into 1-inch pieces and place in a small mixing bowl. Add onion, garlic, ginger, baking soda, cornstarch, and soy sauce, stir together well so that all of the pork is completely covered. Cover and let marinate overnight in refrigerator. When ready to cook, add ¼ cup cornstarch to pork mixture and stir together well, let rest for 5 minutes. Spread remaining cornstarch in a shallow bowl and set aside. Heat 2-3 inches oil in a skillet or fryer on medium heat to 350 degrees. Coat pork pieces individually in cornstarch, pile onto a plate. Fry pork in batches for about 3-4 minutes until golden, transfer to a rack. Fry pork again, starting with the coolest batch for another 1-2 minutes or until pork is a deep golden brown and crispy. Transfer to a rack or plate lined with paper towels. In a small saucepan, combine sugar, vinegar, pineapple juice, ketchup, Worcestershire, soy sauce and cornstarch, whisk together. Turn on heat to medium, whisk in water and cook for about 5 minutes or until it thickens. Transfer pork to a medium size mixing bowl, add thickened sauce and quick toss to coat. Serve immediately with rice and veggies.

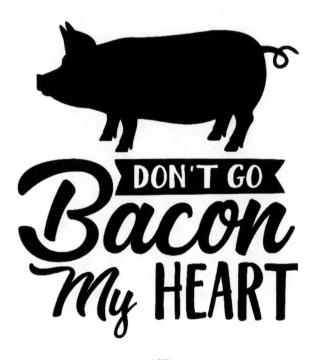

DON'T GO
Bacon
My HEART

Cuban Sandwiches 🍴 *(4 servings)*

For the Pork
2 tbsp. olive oil
2 tbsp. orange juice
1 tbsp. lime juice
1 tbsp. light brown sugar
2 tsp. salt
½ tsp. pepper
½ tsp. paprika
½ tsp. cumin
¼ tsp. garlic powder
1 lb. pork tenderloin

For the Sandwiches
4 gluten-free hoagie rolls
½ cup butter, softened
½ cup yellow mustard
1 lb. deli sliced honey ham
4 large dill pickles, sliced crosswise
16 slices Swiss cheese

Preheat oven to 450 degrees, line a baking sheet with foil. Combine oil, juices, sugar, and seasonings in a small bowl and whisk together well. Add pork tenderloin to a zipper freezer bag and pour in marinade. Seal bag tightly, massage to make sure meat is completely covered. Let marinate at room temperature for about 30 minutes. Transfer tenderloin to baking sheet and pour marinade over top, place pan in oven to roast for about 20-25 minutes or until internal thermometer reads 145 degrees. Transfer to a cutting board and let rest for 5 minutes, then slice into ¼ inch thick pieces.

Slice hoagie rolls lengthwise, spread 1 tbsp. softened butter on the outside of each side of roll. Arrange butter-side down on a cutting board. Spread 1 tbsp. mustard on the inside of each piece of bread. On the bottom layer of bread, layer ¼ amount of ham followed by ¼ amount of pickle slices, ¼ of roasted pork and 2 slices Swiss cheese. Place tops of bread on cheese. Heat a panini maker according to directions. Working in batches, press sandwiches until golden brown and cheese is melted, about 5-6 minutes. Transfer to a cutting board and slice in half diagonally, serve warm.

Grilled Pork Tenderloin 🍴 *(4-6 servings)*

1 1/2 -2 lbs. pork tenderloin
2 tbsp. lemon juice
1 tsp. Italian seasoning
¼ cup olive oil

½ tsp. salt
1/8 tsp. black pepper
1 tbsp. Dijon mustard
1 tbsp. honey

Using paper towels, pat pork tenderloin dry. In a small bowl, combine lemon juice, Italian seasoning, oil, salt, pepper, mustard, and honey, whisk together well. Pour half of marinade into a large zipper freezer bag, add pork, seal bag and massage so that the meat is covered entirely. Let marinate for at least 30 minutes. Preheat grill to medium heat and oil to grates to keep pork from sticking. Using tongs, transfer pork to grill, close and cook for 15-20 minutes. Turn every few minutes to ensure even cooking, brush half of remaining marinade on pork throughout the cooking process. Remove from grill when internal temperature reaches 145 degrees, transfer to a cutting board and let rest for 5 minutes before slicing and serve warm.

Ham and Swiss Mac 'n Cheese ⅱ *(8-10 servings)*

½ cup unsalted butter
½ cup gluten-free all-purpose flour (no XG)
1 tablespoon Dijon mustard
5 cups whole milk
½ tablespoon kosher salt

12 oz. grated Swiss cheese
12 oz. grated white cheddar cheese
1 lb. cubed ham
1 lb. gluten-free elbow pasta
1 lb. grated mozzarella cheese

Preheat oven to 350 degrees. In a large pot, melt butter on medium heat. Whisk in flour and cook for about 1 minute, then add Dijon mustard and whisk again. Slowly pour in milk, whisking well. While the sauce is cooking, stir occasionally. Bring salted water to a boil in another pot. Cook pasta according to package directions for al dente, drain. After sauce has been cooking for about 10-15 minutes and has thickened, turn heat to low and slowly stir in grated cheeses. Stir until melted, remove pot from heat, stir in ham and pasta. Spread into a greased 9x13 inch baking dish, top with grated mozzarella cheese. Bake in oven for 30-40 minutes, or until hot.

Italian Sausage Risotto ⅱ *(4-6 servings)*

1 lb. cooked Italian sausage links
¼ cup butter, divided
8 oz. white mushrooms, sliced
1 clove garlic, minced
½ small onion, diced
1 ½ cups arborio rice

½ cup dry white wine
5 cups chicken broth
1 cup frozen green peas, thawed
2 tsp. Italian seasoning
½ cup freshly grated Parmesan

Slice sausage into ½ inch coins, then quarters, and set aside. Melt 2 tbsp. butter in a large skillet on medium heat and add mushrooms. Cook and stir until soft, about 3-4 minutes. Transfer mushrooms and liquid to a bowl and set aside. Heat remaining butter to skillet, add garlic and onion, cook for 1 minute. Add rice, cook and stir for about 2 minutes, until golden. Add wine and stir constantly until wine is fully absorbed. Add ½ cup broth and stir until absorbed. Continue process with remaining broth, ½ cup at a time and stirring constantly, about 15 minutes until liquid is absorbed and rice is tender. Turn off heat, add peas, Italian seasoning, parmesan, and sausage. Cover and stir until hot, about 3-4 minutes. Serve immediately.

Jambalaya ♈ (4-6 servings)

2 tbsp. canola oil
2 tbsp. Cajun seasoning, divided
1 lb. chicken breast, cut into bite size pieces
12 oz. andouille sausage
1 onion, diced
1 green bell pepper, seeded and diced
2 stalks celery, diced
2 cloves garlic, diced

16 oz. can crushed tomatoes
½ tsp. red pepper flakes
½ tsp. black pepper
1 tsp. salt
½ tsp. hot sauce
2 tsp. gluten-free Worcestershire sauce
1 ¼ cups uncooked white rice
2 ½ cups chicken broth

Heat oil in a large pot or Dutch oven on medium heat. Sprinkle 1 tbsp. Cajun seasoning with chicken, toss to coat. Add chicken to pot and cook until lightly browned, remove from pot using a slotted spoon and set aside. Slice sausage into ½ inch rounds and sprinkle remaining Cajun seasoning all over, toss together before throwing into the pot. Cook sausage until lightly browned on all sides, remove from pot using a slotted spoon and set aside with cooked chicken. Sauté the onion, bell pepper, and celery in pot until tender. Add garlic and cook for 1 minute, just until fragrant. Stir in crushed tomatoes, crushed red pepper, black pepper, salt, hot sauce, and Worcestershire. Add chicken and sausage, cook for 10 minutes while stirring occasionally. Stir in uncooked rice and chicken broth, bring to a boil, then reduce heat and simmer for about 20 minutes or until liquid is absorbed and rice is tender. Serve warm.

Marinated Pork Chops ♈ (6 servings)

6 boneless pork chops (1 inch thick)
1/3 cup olive oil
1/3 cup lemon juice

1/3 cup gluten-free soy sauce
2 tbsp. light brown sugar
2 cloves garlic, minced

Remove pork chops from package and place in a resealable gallon freezer bag. In a small mixing bowl, whisk together remaining ingredients. Pour marinade into bag with pork chops, seal bag and place in refrigerator to marinate for at least one hour. Preheat oven to 375 degrees. Transfer pork chops and marinade to a 9x13 inch baking dish. Cook for about 30 minutes, until meat thermometer reads at least 145 degrees. Serve warm.

Pro-Tip: marinating meat gives it more flavor and moisture, so don't be afraid to let that meat marinate for several hours, or even overnight!

Open-Faced Hamiltons *(4 servings)*

4 gluten-free hamburger buns
16 slices deli ham
2 cups grated extra sharp cheddar cheese
8 oz. cream cheese, softened

½ cup mayonnaise
4 oz. jar pimentos, drained
1/3 cup real bacon bits

Preheat oven to 350 degrees. Slice hamburger buns and lay on a baking sheet, sliced side up. Lay 2 slices of ham on top of each piece of bread. In a medium size mixing bowl, combine cheddar cheese, cream cheese, mayonnaise, drained pimentos, and bacon bits. Using an electric mixer, beat at medium speed until well combined. Scoop about ¼ cup mixture on top of each piece of bread. Place baking sheet in oven and bake for 5-10 minutes, until warm. Serve immediately. If you prefer a cold sandwich, skip the baking process completely and serve cold. Store any leftover **Pimento Cheese** in refrigerator for up to 7 days.

Open-Faced Reubens *(4 servings)*

4 gluten-free hamburger buns
16 slices deli-style corned beef
8 slices Swiss cheese

2 cups sauerkraut
Thousand Island Dressing (p. 99)

Preheat oven to 350 degrees. Slice hamburger buns and lay on a baking sheet, place sliced side up and spread 1 tbsp. dressing on each piece. Lay 2 slices of beef on top and top with a slice of cheese. Place baking sheet in oven for 5-10 minutes, bake until cheese is melted. Remove baking sheet from oven, top each piece with ¼ cup sauerkraut and serve warm.

Pro-Tip: make these Southern-Style **Open-Faced Carolina Reubens** by using turkey to replace beef, and coleslaw to replace sauerkraut!

Parmesan Crusted Pork Chops *(4 servings)*

4 boneless pork chops (1 inch thick)
2 tbsp. mayonnaise

¼ cup grated Parmesan cheese
2 tbsp. gluten-free seasoned breadcrumbs

Preheat oven to 375 degrees. Lay pork chops in a 9x13 inch baking dish. On each pork chop, spread ½ tablespoon mayonnaise on top. Sprinkle 1 tablespoon parmesan on each piece, followed by ½ tablespoon breadcrumbs. Place baking dish in oven and bake for 30-35 minutes, until pork chops are cooked to an internal temperature of at least 145 degrees, and tops are lightly browned. Serve warm.

Pizza Casserole *(4-6 servings)*

4 oz. cream cheese, softened
4 large eggs
1/3 cup heavy cream
¼ cup grated Parmesan cheese
1 clove garlic, minced

½ tsp. Italian seasoning
1 cup grated Romano cheese
2 cups grated mozzarella cheese, divided
½ cup pizza sauce
Pizza toppings of your choice

Preheat oven to 350 degrees, grease a 9x13 inch baking dish with cooking spray and set aside. Combine cream cheese, eggs, heavy cream, parmesan cheese, garlic, and Italian seasoning in a medium size mixing bowl. Beat with electric mixer at medium speed until well combined. Sprinkle Romano and 1 cup mozzarella cheeses into the baking dish, then pour egg mixture on top. Bake in oven for 30 minutes, remove. Spread pizza sauce on top, along with remaining mozzarella and other desired pizza toppings. Set oven to broil on high, then place baking dish back in oven until it becomes brown and bubbly. Remove from oven, let sit for a few minutes before slicing.

Pork Medallions *(4-6 servings)*

1 tsp. paprika
1 tsp. garlic powder
1 tsp. onion powder
1 tsp. Italian seasoning
½ tsp. salt

½ tsp. pepper
2 pork tenderloins
2 tbsp. olive oil
½ cup chicken bone broth
2 tbsp. butter

In a small bowl, combine paprika, garlic powder, onion powder, Italian seasoning, salt, and pepper, whisk together and set aside. Cut each tenderloin into 12 slices and pat them dry with paper towels. Lay on a baking sheet and sprinkle seasoning mixture on both sides of each medallion. Heat olive oil in a large skillet pan on medium/high heat, sear medallions on each side for 2-3 minutes. You will cook the medallions in two batches, so feel free to add more olive oil for the second batch if needed. Remove medallions from pan and add bone broth, scraping pan to remove bits. Add butter and whisk until melted, remove pan from heat and add medallions back to pan to coat them completely. Serve warm.

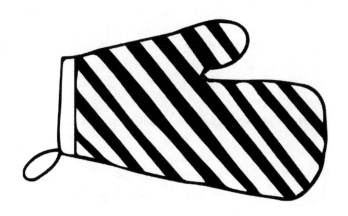

Pork Milanese ⚲ (6 servings)

1 cup gluten-free breadcrumbs
½ freshly grated parmesan cheese
2 large eggs
6 boneless pork chops

Salt and pepper, to taste
½ cup olive oil
1 lemon

Combine breadcrumbs and parmesan cheese in a shallow bowl, toss together and set aside. Beat eggs in a separate shallow bowl, set aside. Lay pork chops on a baking sheet and sprinkle each side with salt and pepper. Heat olive oil in a large skillet on medium heat. Dip each pork chop in beaten eggs, then in breadcrumb mixture to evenly coat on each side. Cook 3 pork chops at a time for about 3 minutes on each side in hot oil until golden brown. Transfer to paper towels to drain, cook remaining pork chops. Slice lemon into 6 wedges, serve with each pork chop and squeeze juice on top.

Pulled Pork ⚲ (8-10 servings)

4 lb. pork shoulder or butt
1 tbsp. light brown sugar
1 tbsp. chili powder
1 tsp. onion powder
1 tsp. garlic powder

1 tsp. ground cumin
1 tsp. salt
1 tsp. black pepper
½ cup apple cider vinegar
½ cup apple juice

Preheat oven to 300 degrees. Trim pork of excess fat and cut into 4 equal size pieces. In a small bowl, combine brown sugar, chili powder, onion powder, garlic powder, cumin, salt, and pepper, stir together well to combine. Rub equally all over pork. In a Dutch Oven pot, place pork inside. Combine apple cider vinegar and apple juice, pour in with pork. Cover with lid and bake in oven for 3 hours. Remove lid and continue cooking for another 1-2 hours, until pork is tender and easily comes apart with a fork. Remove pot from oven, shred meat and add barbecue sauce if desired.

⚲ **Pro-Tip:** make **Pork Tacos** for dinner! Load up your corn or gluten-free tortillas with pork, top with BBQ sauce, pico de gallo, and coleslaw for a little twist on Taco Tuesday.

Make this in a slow cooker using the same process but cook on low for 3-4 hours!

Ravioli Lasagna ⚱ *(6-8 servings)*

30 oz. frozen gluten-free cheese ravioli

2 (24 oz.) jars spaghetti sauce

16 oz. ricotta cheese, at room temp

2 (4 oz.) packages cooked sausage crumbles*

¾ cup grated Parmesan cheese

4 cups grated mozzarella cheese

Preheat oven to 375 degrees. Cook ravioli according to package directions, drain and set aside. Coat a 9x13 inch baking dish with cooking spray. Spread half of 1 jar spaghetti sauce on the bottom of baking dish. Place one layer of ravioli on top of spaghetti sauce. Spread half of ricotta on top of ravioli (don't worry about it being in an even layer or even being pretty, no one will care what it looks like when they take a bite). Pour other half of spaghetti sauce on top of ricotta layer. Sprinkle 1 package of sausage crumbles on top, followed by ¼ cup Parmesan cheese and 1 cup mozzarella cheese. Repeat layering. For top layer, place remaining ravioli on top, remaining spaghetti sauce, Parmesan and mozzarella. Bake for 35 minutes. Remove from oven and let sit for 10 minutes before serving.

⚱ **Pro-Tip:** if cooked sausage crumbles aren't available in your grocery store (found with sausage in the refrigerated section), you can use ground sausage instead. Cook the sausage in a skillet until browned and fully cooked, drain liquid and use in recipe.

Smothered Pork Chops with Gravy ⚱ *(4-6 servings)*

4-6 thick cut boneless pork chops

¼ cup olive oil

½ cup gluten-free all-purpose flour (no XG)

1 tbsp. onion powder

1 cup chicken broth

10 oz. gluten-free cream of mushroom soup

Pat pork chops dry with paper towel, set aside. Heat olive oil in skillet on medium heat. In a bowl, whisk together flour and onion powder. When oil is hot, dredge each pork chop in flour on both sides, place in hot oil in pan. Cook on each side for 2-3 minutes, until a light golden color. Remove pork chops from pan and set aside on plate. Reduce heat to low/medium, whisk in 2 tablespoons of flour mixture you used for dredging the pork chops. Cook for 1 minute and slowly whisk in chicken broth. Stir until ingredients are combined, then add cream of mushroom soup. Whisk again, place pork chops back in pan with gravy and cover. Cook for about 10 minutes, until pork chops are cooked through. Serve warm. This gravy goes well over rice or mashed potatoes.

Southern BBQ Casserole (6-8 servings)

1 lb. cooked pulled pork
28 oz. can gluten-free baked beans
8 oz. gluten-free elbow pasta
1 cup mayonnaise

1 cup sour cream
4 cups grated sharp cheddar cheese
½ cup butter, melted

Preheat oven to 350 degrees. If pork is vacuum-sealed, pull apart to loosen before putting in the bottom of a greased 9x13 inch baking dish in an even layer. Spoon baked beans on top. In a pot, cook pasta according to package directions for al dente, drain and set aside. In a large mixing bowl, whisk together mayonnaise and sour cream. Add pasta, 3 cups cheddar cheese, and parmesan; stir together well. Spoon the macaroni on top of baked beans, sprinkle with remaining cheddar cheese and drizzle with melted butter. Bake for 30-40 minutes, until hot and cheese is melted. Serve warm.

Stuffed Pork Tenderloin (4-6 servings)

¼ cup olive oil, divided
2 slices bacon, diced
6 oz. sliced mushrooms
½ small onion, diced
½ tbsp. salt, divided

½ tsp. pepper, divided
1 clove garlic, minced
¼ cup fresh parsley, chopped
1 ½ lb. pork tenderloin

Preheat oven to 400 degrees. Heat an oven-safe large skillet over medium heat. Add 2 tbsp. olive oil and chopped bacon, cook until browned, about 3-4 minutes. Add mushrooms and onion, sauté for 5 minutes or until tender. Stir in ½ tsp. salt, ¼ tsp. pepper, garlic, and parsley, cook for another minute before transferring to a bowl. Remove silver skin from pork tenderloin, then cut a slit all the way down the long end but do not cut all the way through. Open tenderloin like a book, then cover with a piece of plastic wrap. Using the flat side of a meat mallet, pound to ½ inch thick without tearing through the meat. Spoon mushroom mixture over tenderloin and spread into an even layer, leaving ½ inch space around the edges. Starting with the long end, roll up tightly and secure the ends with 6-8 toothpicks. Make sure to stick toothpicks through to create a flat cooking surface for the bottom. Sprinkle remaining salt and pepper all over tenderloin. Bring the same skillet back to medium heat and add remaining 2 tbsp. olive oil. When oil is hot, place the tenderloin toothpick side down into skillet to sear for 2 minutes on all four sides. Transfer skillet with the tenderloin to the preheated oven and bake for 18-20 minutes or until the thickest part of the meat is 145 degrees. Transfer tenderloin to a cutting board, let rest for 10 minutes. Brush pan drippings on top and slice into 1-inch pieces. Serve warm.

Baked Red Snapper 🍷 *(4 servings)*

4 (6-8 oz) red snapper fillets
½ cup butter
2 cloves garlic, minced
1 tsp. gluten-free Worcestershire sauce
1 tsp. Cajun seasoning

¼ tsp. black pepper
1 tsp. dried parsley
½ cup gluten-free breadcrumbs
¼ cup freshly grated parmesan cheese

Preheat oven to 400 degrees, coat a baking dish with cooking spray and place fillets skin-side down in dish. In a small saucepan, melt butter on medium heat, add garlic, Worcestershire sauce, Cajun seasoning, pepper, and parsley. Cook on low heat for 2 minutes just to blend flavors, then brush both sides of each fillet with sauce. In a small bowl, combine breadcrumbs and parmesan cheese, toss together. Distribute breadcrumb mixture evenly on top of each fillet and press down. Place dish in oven and bake for about 12 minutes (depending on thickness of fillets), just until opaque and flake easily with a fork. Serve warm.

I Have It All TOGETHER (I JUST) FORGOT =where= I PUT IT

Bang Bang Shrimp *(4 servings)*

½ cup mayonnaise
¼ cup Thai sweet chili sauce
¼ tsp. sriracha
1 lb. shrimp, peeled and deveined (no tails)

½ cup buttermilk
¾ cup cornstarch
Canola oil (for frying)

In a small bowl, combine mayonnaise, sweet chili sauce, and sriracha, stir together well then set aside. In a small mixing bowl, combine shrimp and buttermilk, stir to coat well. Let shrimp sit for about 10 minutes. Pour shrimp and buttermilk into a strainer to remove buttermilk from shrimp. In a medium size mixing bowl, combine shrimp and cornstarch, toss together well to coat completely. In a heavy bottom pan or fryer, heat at least 2-3 inches canola oil to 375 degrees. When oil is hot, fry the shrimp until golden brown, about 1-2 minutes on each side. Transfer to paper towels to drain excess oil, then immediately toss together with sauce and serve.

Coconut Shrimp *(4 servings)*

1/3 cup gluten-free all-purpose flour
½ tsp. salt
½ tsp. pepper
2 large eggs
¾ cup gluten-free panko breadcrumbs

1 cup sweetened shredded coconut
1 lb. shrimp, peeled and deveined (with tails)
Canola oil (for frying)
3 tbsp. Thai sweet chili sauce
6 tbsp. orange or apricot jam or preserves

In one bowl, combine flour, salt, and pepper, whisk together and set aside. In a second bowl, beat eggs. In a third bowl, combine breadcrumbs and coconut, toss together. Dip shrimp into flour, then eggs, then dredge in coconut mixture and press gently to help stick. You want a lot of the coconut mixture on each piece of shrimp. Set coated shrimp aside on parchment paper and continue process until all of them are finished. In a heavy bottom pan or fryer, heat at least 2-3 inches canola oil to 375 degrees. When oil is hot, fry the shrimp until golden brown, about 1-2 minutes on each side, then transfer to paper towels to drain excess oil. In a small bowl, combine chili sauce and jam, whisk together well and serve as a dipping sauce for shrimp.

These two recipes are a couple of mine and my husband's favorites when we go out to particular restaurants. Although I "think" the Bang Bang Shrimp is gluten-free, there are no guarantees when you order from a restaurant and the server doesn't even know what gluten is. Traditional Coconut Shrimp is definitely not gluten-free, so this is a must-have recipe for making it at home.

Crab Cakes ⚔ *(4-6 servings)*

For the Crab Cakes
¼ cup mayonnaise
1 egg, beaten
2 tsp. dried parsley
2 tsp. Dijon mustard
2 tsp. gluten-free Worcestershire
1 lb. lump crab meat, drained
2/3 cup gluten-free panko breadcrumbs

For the Remoulade
1 cup mayonnaise
1 ½ tbsp. sweet relish
1 tsp. Dijon mustard
½ tsp. onion powder
1-2 tbsp. lemon juice
Sea salt (to taste)

Preheat oven to 450 degrees. In a medium size mixing bowl, whisk together the mayonnaise, egg, parsley, mustard, and Worcestershire. Add crab meat and breadcrumbs, stir together well. Form into 6 hockey puck shaped patties and place on an aluminum-lined pan, place in refrigerator for about 20 minutes to set. Remove from fridge, roll in more breadcrumbs (if desired) and bake for 15-18 minutes, until lightly browned and crispy. While Crab Cakes are baking, make the sauce. Combine all ingredients in a small mixing bowl and whisk together well. Serve with crab cakes drizzled on top or on the side to dip.

Crab Fritters ⚔ *(4-6 servings)*

For the Dipping Sauce
¾ cup mayonnaise
1 tbsp. Dijon mustard
1 tbsp. horseradish
2 cloves garlic, minced
2 tbsp. lemon juice
1 tbsp. chopped fresh chives

For the Fritters
canola oil (for frying)
1 batch Hush Puppies Batter (p. 27)
1 lb. cooked lump crabmeat

Combine all ingredients for dipping sauce and whisk together well, set aside in refrigerator while preparing fritters. Heat 3-4 inches oil in a heavy bottomed pot or fryer to 375 degrees. Prepare fritters using Hush Puppies recipe, stir in crabmeat. Drop 1 tablespoon at a time into hot oil and fry until golden brown, about 2-3 minutes. Transfer to paper towels to catch excess grease, serve warm with prepared dipping sauce.

Deep-Fried Catfish Fillets 🍴 *(4 servings)*

4 catfish fillets (about 1 lb.)
1 cup buttermilk
2 cups gluten-free cornmeal
1 tbsp. cayenne pepper

1 tsp. salt
1 tsp. pepper
Canola oil, for frying
Tartar Sauce (p. 90)

Using paper towels, pat fillets dry. Place fillets in a bowl with buttermilk, making sure they are completely immersed and let sit for 10 minutes in refrigerator. In a medium size mixing bowl, combine cornmeal, cayenne, salt, and pepper, whisk together well. Heat oil (at least 2-3 inches deep) in a Dutch oven or fryer to 350 degrees. Remove fillets one at a time from buttermilk, coating in cornmeal mixture on both sides. Repeat process again, then cook 2 fillets at a time when the oil is ready. Fry for 2 ½ - 3 minutes on each side, do not turn over until done cooking on each side. Internal temperature should be 145 degrees, repeat cooking process with remaining 2 fillets. Place fillets on paper towels to catch excess grease, serve with Tartar Sauce (p. 90).

Fish Sticks 🍴 *(4 servings)*

1 ½ lbs. cod fillets, skin removed
Salt and pepper to taste
1 tsp. black pepper
1 tsp. dried oregano
1 tsp. paprika

½ cup gluten-free all-purpose flour
2 large eggs + 1 tbsp. water
½ cup gluten-free breadcrumbs
½ cup freshly grated parmesan
1 lemon

Preheat oven to 450 degrees. Pat fillets dry with paper towel, then season with salt and pepper on both sides. Cut into sticks that are about 1-1/2 inches thick by 3 inches long and set aside. In a shallow bowl, combine black pepper, oregano, paprika, and flour, whisk together. In a second shallow bowl, beat eggs with 1 tbsp. water. In a third bowl, combine breadcrumbs, parmesan, and zest from lemon. Toss together well and set aside. Take each fish stick and dredge in flour mixture, then egg mixture, and breadcrumb mixture. Gently pat each fish stick to make sure the breadcrumb mixture sticks. Grease a baking sheet with cooking spray and arrange fish sticks on sheet, spray the tops of fish sticks with a little more cooking spray. Bake in preheated oven for 12-15 minutes or until a light golden brown. Drizzle with juice from lemon, if desired and serve warm with your choice of sauce for dipping (remoulade, tartar, ketchup, etc.).

Fish Tacos 🍴 *(8-10 servings)*

For the Fish
1 ½ lbs. tilapia
½ tsp. ground cumin
½ tsp. cayenne pepper
1 tsp. salt
¼ tsp. black pepper
2 tbsp. olive oil

For the Sauce
½ cup sour cream
½ cup mayonnaise
2 tbsp. lime juice
1 tsp. garlic powder
1 tsp. sriracha sauce

For the Tacos
Gluten-free or corn tortillas
Shredded cabbage or lettuce
2 avocados, pitted and sliced

Prepared pico de gallo
Grated pepper jack cheese

Preheat oven to 375 degrees, line a large baking sheet with parchment paper, lay tilapia on top and set aside. In a small bowl, combine cumin, cayenne, salt, and pepper, stir together and sprinkle on each side of tilapia. Lightly drizzle with olive oil and bake for about 25 minutes. To make the sauce, combine all ingredients in a bowl, whisk together and set aside. Pull apart fish to prepare tacos. To assemble, start with fish, then add desired remaining ingredients and serve immediately.

Gourmet Lobster Mac 'n Cheese 🍴 *(6-8 servings)*

½ cup butter
½ cup gluten-free all-purpose flour (no XG)
3 ½ cups whole milk
1 cup heavy cream
1 tbsp. Dijon mustard
1 tsp. salt

¼ tsp. black pepper
8 oz. white cheddar cheese, grated
8 oz. gruyere cheese, grated
1 lb. sharp cheddar cheese, grated
1 lb. gluten-free pasta (penne or elbow)
1 lb. frozen cooked lobster, thawed

Preheat oven to 350 degrees. In a stock pot, melt butter on medium heat. Whisk in flour and cook for about 1 minute. Slowly pour in milk, heavy cream, and Dijon mustard, whisking well. While the sauce is cooking, bring salted water to a boil in another pot. Cook pasta according to package directions, only to al dente (if the pasta is cooked too much, it can get mushy in the sauce after it sits), drain pasta and set aside. After sauce has been cooking for about 10-15 minutes and has thickened, turn heat to low and slowly stir in grated cheeses, salt and pepper. Stir until melted, remove pot from heat, stir in lobster and pasta. Spread into a greased 9x13 inch baking dish and top with extra grated cheddar cheese, if desired. Bake in oven for 30-40 minutes, until hot and bubbly. Remove from oven, let sit for 5-10 minutes before serving.

Grouper Fromage (8-10 servings)

2 tbsp. butter
1 small onion, diced
1 tsp. seasoned salt, divided
1 tsp. hot sauce
1 cup mayonnaise

2 cups grated Monterey Jack cheese
4 (8 oz.) grouper fillets
1 tsp. red pepper flakes
1 lemon, halved
¼ cup butter

Preheat oven to 350 degrees. Melt butter in a small skillet, add onion and cook until softened, stirring occasionally. Transfer to a medium size mixing bowl to cool slightly. Add ½ tsp. seasoned salt, hot sauce, mayonnaise, and cheese, stir together and set aside. Grease a 9x13 inch baking dish with cooking spray, lay fillets inside dish, sprinkle with red pepper flakes and drizzle with ½ of lemon juice. Slice butter into 4 pieces, place one piece on top of each fillet. Place dish in oven to bake for about 15 minutes, until fish is almost done. Remove from oven, cover fillets with cheese mixture, return to oven to bake again for 8-10 minutes. Serve warm.

Low Country Boil (14-16 servings)

1 tbsp. seafood seasoning (like Old Bay)
5 lbs. new potatoes, halved
3 (16 oz.) packaged kielbasa sausages

8 ears fresh corn
5 lbs. whole crab, broken into pieces
4 lbs. fresh shrimp, peeled and deveined

Heat a very large pot of water over medium/high heat, add seasoning and bring to a boil. Add potatoes and sausage, cook for 10 minutes. Cut each ear of corn into 2 or 3 equal size pieces, add to pot along with crab. Cook for another 5 minutes. When potatoes are almost tender and everything else is almost done, add shrimp and cook for another 3-4 minutes, just until they're cooked through. Drain and discard water, pour into large foil pans for serving.

Open-Faced Crab Avocado Sandwiches (2-4 servings)

4 slices gluten-free bread
1 ripe avocado, peeled and sliced
8 oz. crab meat, drained
2 tbsp. mayonnaise

1 tsp. Dijon mustard
1 tbsp. lemon juice
2 tsp. chopped fresh dill
Salt and pepper to taste

Place bread in toaster and toast until golden, set on plates. Lay avocado slices on top of each piece of bread. In a small bowl, combine crab meat, mayonnaise, mustard, lemon juice, fresh dill, and a light sprinkle of salt and pepper. Stir to combine, then spoon equally on top of bread slices and serve immediately.

Roasted Shrimp with Peanut Sauce *(4-6 servings)*

2 lbs. shrimp, peeled and deveined
1 tbsp. olive oil
½ tsp. salt
½ tsp. pepper
½ cup creamy peanut butter
2 tbsp. gluten-free soy sauce
1 tbsp. rice vinegar

2 tbsp. light brown sugar
2 tsp. chili sauce
1 tbsp. lime juice
3 garlic cloves, minced
1 tbsp. grated ginger
2-4 tbsp. warm water

Preheat oven to 400 degrees. Leave tails on the shrimp, combine with olive oil in a medium size mixing bowl and gently toss together to coat evenly. Grease a baking sheet with cooking spray, spread shrimp on pan and sprinkle with salt and pepper. Roast for 8-10 minutes, just until pink and cooked through. While the shrimp is roasting, make the sauce. In a small mixing bowl, combine peanut butter, soy sauce, rice vinegar, sugar, chili sauce, lime juice, garlic, and ginger, whisk together well. Add water 1 tbsp. at a time to reach desired consistency. Serve with warm shrimp.

Salmon Patties *(4 servings)*

2 (6 oz.) cans boneless skinless salmon
2 large eggs, beaten
2 tbsp. mayonnaise
2 tsp. Dijon mustard
1 clove garlic, minced

½ tsp. salt
¼ tsp. pepper
½ tsp. dried thyme
½ cup chopped parsley
¼ cup coconut or avocado oil

Drain salmon thoroughly before placing in a medium size mixing bowl. Using a fork, flake it into tiny pieces. Add eggs, mayonnaise, mustard, garlic, salt, pepper, and thyme, mix well. Add chopped parsley and stir together. Heat oil in a 12-inch skillet on medium heat. When oil is hot, use an ice cream scoop to scoop out crab mixture into oil and gently flatten using a spatula. You should be able to cook 4 patties at one time. Cook until browned and crispy, about 3 minutes on each side. Transfer to a plate lined with paper towels to catch excess grease, serve warm.

Sauteed Shrimp *(4-6 servings)*

1 lb. fresh shrimp, peeled and de-veined
2 tsp. Italian seasoning
½ tsp. salt
1 tsp. paprika

¼ tsp. ground black pepper
4 tbsp. unsalted butter
1 oz. white wine or cooking sherry
1 clove garlic, minced

Toss together shrimp and dry seasonings in a small mixing bowl. Melt butter in pan on medium heat, add wine and garlic. Continue cooking for 1 minute, then add shrimp. Cook shrimp until opaque and cooked through, about 2-4 minutes. Serve warm.

Seafood Casserole 🍴 *(6-8 servings)*

1 cup uncooked white rice + 2 cups water
2 tbsp. butter
2 celery ribs, diced
½ onion, diced
6 oz. sliced mushrooms
2 tbsp. diced pimentos
1 lb. can lump crab meat, drained

1 lb. frozen cooked shrimp, thawed
8 oz. sour cream
1 cup milk
½ tsp. black pepper
1 ½ tsp. salt
1 cup gluten-free breadcrumbs
½ cup butter, melted

Preheat oven to 350 degrees. Cook rice according to package directions. While rice is cooking, melt butter in a skillet pan and sauté celery, onions, and mushrooms until veggies are tender, pour into a large mixing bowl. Add cooked rice, shrimp, crab, and pimentos. Stir together well. In a medium size mixing bowl, whisk together the sour cream, milk, salt, and pepper. Pour into large bowl with other ingredients and stir together well, then spread into a greased 9x13 inch baking dish. In a small mixing bowl, toss together breadcrumbs and butter, sprinkle on top. Bake in oven for 35-45 minutes, until hot.

Shrimp and Grits 🍴 *(4-6 servings)*

2 pieces thick cut bacon, cut into bite size pieces
1 tbsp. unsalted butter
1 lb. fresh shrimp, peeled and de-veined
¼ cup cooking sherry or white wine
½ cup heavy cream
¼ cup roasted red bell pepper, minced

2 green onions, minced
1 tsp. BBQ seasoning
½ teaspoon sugar
½ tsp. salt
½ cup freshly grated parmesan

In a large skillet on medium heat, cook bacon until crispy. Remove bacon from pan and set aside, leaving bacon fat in pan. Add butter and stir until melted, then add shrimp. Sauté until opaque and tender. Add wine and cook for another 1-2 minutes, until sauce slightly reduces. Stir in heavy cream, bell pepper, green onions, BBQ seasoning, sugar, and salt. Cook for another 2-3 minutes, add parmesan cheese and stir. Cook for another 2-3 minutes until sauce has thickened. Spoon shrimp and sauce over grits.

Shrimp Diablo 🍴 *(4 servings)*

½ tbsp. olive oil
1 small onion, diced
2 cloves garlic, minced
14.5 oz. can fire roasted diced tomatoes
¼ cup chopped cilantro

1 tbsp. chopped chipotle in adobo
1 tsp. light brown sugar
½ tsp. salt
1 lb. peeled and deveined shrimp (no tails)

Heat oil in a large skillet pan on medium heat, add onion and sauté for 3-4 minutes or until tender and translucent. Add garlic and sauté for another 30 seconds, then transfer to a blender. Add tomatoes, cilantro, chipotle in adobo, brown sugar, and salt. Puree until smooth. Transfer sauce back to skillet, add shrimp and stir together. Let shrimp cook in sauce for about 5 minutes, or until shrimp are cooked and sauce has slightly thickened. Serve warm with Mexican Rice (p. 189), roasted vegetables, in fajitas or tacos.

Shrimp Skewers 🍴 *(6-8 servings)*

6 tbsp. olive oil
4 tbsp. lemon juice
1 tsp. salt
½ tsp. black pepper

1 tsp. dried oregano
1 tsp. paprika
1 tsp. garlic powder
2 lbs. peeled and deveined shrimp

Place wooden skewers in water to soak while preparing shrimp (this will keep the skewers from burning on the grill). In a medium size mixing bowl, combine olive oil, lemon juice, salt, pepper, oregano, paprika, and garlic powder, whisk together well and set aside. Add shrimp to bowl, toss to coat completely and let shrimp marinate for at least 15 minutes, 2 hours max. Remove skewers from water and skewer 4-6 shrimp on each one, place on a plate until ready to cook. Heat a grill or grill pan on medium/high heat, cook shrimp for 2-3 minutes on each side until the color is pink and shrimp is opaque. Serve warm.

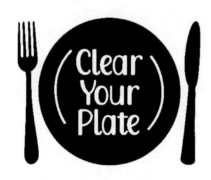

Southern Shrimp and Pasta 🍴 *(6-8 servings)*

1 cup butter
1 cup gluten-free all-purpose flour (no XG)
1 cup white wine or cooking sherry
1 tbsp. BBQ seasoning
5 cups half and half
1 lb. frozen cooked shrimp, thawed

1 lb. gluten-free penne pasta
2 green onions, minced
½ cup real bacon bits
½ cup roasted red bell pepper, diced
1-2 tsp. salt
1 lb. grated mozzarella cheese

Preheat oven to 350 degrees. Melt butter in a pot on medium heat until melted, whisk in flour. Slowly add sherry and BBQ seasoning, whisk and continue to cook for another minute. Whisk in half and half, continue to cook on medium heat, whisking occasionally to break up any clumps from the roux (the butter and flour mixture). While the sauce is cooking, cook the pasta according to package directions just until al dente. So, if the package directions say 8-10 minutes, pull the pasta off the stove right at 8 minutes, pour into strainer and run cold water over the pasta to stop it from cooking; set aside. When the sauce has been cooking for about 12-15 minutes and has thickened, remove from heat and stir in shrimp, green onions, bacon, roasted red bell peppers, and salt. Spread into a greased 9x13 inch baking dish sprinkle with mozzarella cheese. Bake in oven for 30-40 minutes, until hot and cheese is melted.

Steamed Lemon Salmon 🍴 *(6-8 servings)*

2 lb. side of salmon
5 sprigs fresh rosemary
2 small lemons, thinly sliced
2 tbsp. olive oil

1 tsp. salt
¼ tsp. black pepper
4 cloves garlic, minced
2 green onions, sliced

Remove salmon from refrigerator and preheat oven to 375 degrees. Line a large baking sheet with aluminum foil and coat with cooking spray. Place 2 sprigs of rosemary down the middle, then slices from 1 lemon. Place salmon on top, drizzle with olive oil and sprinkle with salt and pepper. Rub to coat well, then sprinkle garlic on top and layer remaining rosemary and lemon slices on top. Fold sides of the foil up and over top of the salmon until it is completely enclosed. If the foil is not large enough to do this, place another piece of foil on top and fold the edges under to form a sealed packet. Leave some room inside foil for air to circulate during the baking process. Bake salmon for 15-20 minutes, until almost cooked completely through the thickest part. Baking time will depend on the thickness of salmon. Remove salmon from oven and carefully open foil so the top is completely uncovered, watch out for a steam cloud! Change setting on oven to broil, then return to oven to broil for 3 minutes until salmon is slightly golden and cooked through. Be careful not to overcook or burn garlic. Remove from oven, cut into portions and garnish with green onions, serve warm.

Teriyaki Salmon ⸙ *(8 servings)*

3 tbsp. gluten-free teriyaki sauce
3 tbsp. gluten-free hoisin sauce
3 tbsp. gluten-free soy sauce
1 tbsp. vinegar
1 tbsp. sesame oil

¼ cup light brown sugar
2 cloves garlic, minced
½ tsp. ground ginger
2 ½ lbs. salmon filet
2 tbsp. sesame seeds

Preheat oven to 400 degrees and line a large, rimmed baking sheet with foil. In a small bowl, combine teriyaki sauce, hoisin sauce, soy sauce, vinegar, sesame oil, sugar, garlic, and ginger, whisk together and set aside. Slice salmon filet into 8 pieces and place in a large zipper freezer bag. Pour half of sauce into bag and seal, massage to make sure all of salmon pieces are coated evenly. Let marinate for 20-30 minutes. Transfer salmon filets to the prepared baking sheet. Bake for 12-16 minutes, or until salmon is flaky and cooked through (bake time may vary depending on thickness of salmon). Pour the remaining marinade into a small saucepan and bring to a boil, then reduce to a simmer until slightly thickened. When salmon is done cooking, brush with sauce and sprinkle with sesame seeds, serve warm.

Tuna Melts ⸙ *(4 servings)*

4 gluten-free hamburger buns
2 (5 oz.) cans tuna packed in water, drained
¼ cup mayonnaise

2 tbsp. relish
½ tsp. seasoned salt
4 slices cheddar cheese

Preheat oven to high broil setting. Slice hamburger buns and lay on a baking sheet, sliced side up. In a small mixing bowl, combine tuna, mayonnaise, relish, and seasoned salt. Stir together well. Spoon evenly over each piece of bread, top with 1 slice of cheese. Place baking sheet in oven, broil for about 2 minutes, or until cheese is melted and edges of bread are slightly toasted. Serve warm.

You know this is an easy recipe when it is made on a regular basis by college students who have no idea how to cook. That was my roommates and myself back in the stone ages, and this was one of our regular meals. I honestly didn't consider this an open-faced sandwich until I learned what an open-faced sandwich was. Eye-opening.

When IN
DOUBT

–ADD–
Bacon

Vegetarian & Side Dishes

Baked Brown Rice 🍴 *(4-6 servings)*

1 ½ cups brown rice
2 ½ cups gluten-free beef broth

2 tbsp. butter

Preheat oven to 375 degrees. Dump the rice into an 8x8 inch baking dish. In a saucepan, bring broth and butter to a boil before pouring over rice in dish. Cover top of dish tightly with aluminum foil, place dish in oven and bake for 1 hour. Remove foil, fluff with a fork and serve warm.

Baked Cheese Tortellini 🍴 *(6-8 servings)*

24 oz. gluten-free cheese tortellini
12 oz. steam-in-a-bag broccoli
24 oz. jar spaghetti sauce

15 oz. jar gluten-free alfredo sauce
½ cup grated parmesan cheese
2 cups grated mozzarella cheese

Preheat oven to 375 degrees. Cook tortellini according to package directions, drain. Coat 9x13 inch baking dish with cooking spray, spoon cooked tortellini in dish. Cook broccoli in microwave, according to package directions. Arrange cooked broccoli on top of tortellini in dish. In a small mixing bowl, stir together both jars of sauce until well combined. Spoon over broccoli and tortellini in baking dish into an even layer. Sprinkle Parmesan cheese on top of sauce, followed by mozzarella cheese. Place dish in oven and bake for 30 minutes. Remove dish from oven and serve warm.

Baked Mac 'n Cheese 🍴🍴 *(14-16 servings)*

16 oz. gluten-free elbow macaroni
½ cup unsalted butter
½ cup gluten-free all-purpose flour (no XG)
1 teaspoon Dijon mustard
1 tsp. salt

½ tsp. pepper
5 cups whole milk
2 lbs. block sharp cheddar
½ cup grated parmesan cheese

Preheat oven to 350 degrees. Cook pasta according to package directions just to al dente, drain and set aside. Melt butter in a pot on medium heat, add flour and Dijon mustard, whisk until smooth and cook for about 1 minute. Slowly add milk to flour mixture, whisking constantly until smooth. Add salt and pepper. Continue to cook on medium heat for 12-15 minutes, or until sauce is thickened, stirring occasionally. While sauce is cooking, grate cheddar cheese. Add cheddar cheese and parmesan cheese, stir again until sauce is smooth and cheeses are melted. Remove sauce from heat and stir in drained pasta. Pour mixture into your greased freezer containers, sprinkle with extra cheddar if desired. Bake in oven for 35-45 minutes, until hot and cheese is melted.

🍴**Pro-Tip:** grating the cheese yourself makes a huge difference in the creamy texture of this recipe. It's not mandatory to grate it yourself, but highly recommended!

Baked Potatoes (4 servings)

4 large baking potatoes
1 tbsp. olive oil

sea salt
¼ cup unsalted butter

Preheat oven to 450 degrees. Scrub potatoes under running water, then dry and rub the skin of each one with oil and sprinkle with salt. Use a fork to pierce the skin evenly around each potato. Place potatoes on a baking pan and bake in oven for 45-60 minutes, depending on the size of your potatoes. When a knife is inserted and no resistance occurs, the potatoes are done. Remove from oven, cut down the middle and serve immediately with butter.

Bean Cakes (4-6 servings)

15 oz. can pinto beans, rinsed and drained
2 tbsp. gluten-free flour

1 tsp. onion powder
¼ cup vegetable oil, for frying

Rinse and drain pinto beans, transfer to a medium size mixing bowl and mash well using a potato masher. Add flour and onion powder, mix well with hands and shape into small patties. Set patties on a parchment paper lined plate or small baking sheet. Heat oil in skillet on medium heat. When oil is hot, place cakes in batches and fry in oil for 3-4 minutes on each side, until browned and crispy. Remove from pan and set on paper towels to catch grease before serving.

Bean Enchiladas (8-10 servings)

15 oz. can black beans, rinsed and drained
29 oz. can refried beans
8 oz. sour cream
1 oz. packet taco seasoning

12-14 gluten-free corn tortillas
2 cups grated Mexican blend cheese
24 oz. salsa or Enchilada Sauce (p. 86)

Preheat oven to 375 degrees. In a medium sized mixing bowl, combine all cans of beans, sour cream, and taco seasoning. Using an electric mixer, beat at medium speed for 1 minute until all ingredients are well combined. Place tortillas on a plate and heat in microwave for 15-20 seconds (warming the tortillas makes them easier to handle). Spread ¼ cup bean mixture into one tortilla along the middle, about 1 inch from two sides. Tuck in the sides and roll up like a burrito. Coat a 9x13 inch baking dish with cooking spray and place each enchilada in baking dish, seam side down. When finished with all enchiladas, pour sauce evenly on top. Sprinkle with cheese and bake for 30-35 minutes, until hot and cheese is melted. Serve warm.

Beans and Brown Rice (10-12 servings)

1 cup brown rice
15 oz. can great northern beans
15 oz. can lima beans

15 oz. can pinto beans
15 oz. can black eyed peas
15 oz. can black beans

Cook brown rice according to package directions. While rice is cooking, open each can of beans and pour into a large strainer. Rinse with cold water, then dump into a medium size pot and add 1 cup of water. Cook on medium heat until beans are hot. When rice is done cooking, remove from heat and transfer to pot with beans, stir together. Serve warm or spoon into microwave safe dishes for a quick and easy lunch.

Black Bean Burgers (4 servings)

15 oz. can refried black beans
½ cup diced onion
½ cup diced bell peppers

1 egg, beaten
1 tbsp. Montreal steak seasoning
¾ cup gluten-free breadcrumbs

Preheat oven to 375 degrees. Open can of refried beans and drain liquid. Scoop beans out of can and into a medium sized mixing bowl. Add remaining ingredients, mix well with hands. Divide into four thick patties about the width of a hamburger bun. Place aluminum foil on a baking sheet and lightly coat with cooking spray. Place patties on baking sheet and bake for 12 minutes on each side. Serve warm on a gluten-free bun with your favorite condiments.

Broccoli Casserole (6-8 servings)

20 oz. frozen chopped broccoli, thawed
10 oz. can gluten-free cream of mushroom soup
1 cup mayonnaise
1 cup grated cheddar cheese

1 egg, beaten
1 tsp. onion powder
½ cup gluten-free breadcrumbs
2 tbsp. butter, melted

Preheat oven to 375 degrees. Drain broccoli and add to a medium size mixing bowl. Add soup, mayonnaise, cheese, egg, and onion powder. Stir together well and spoon into a greased 8x8 inch baking dish. Sprinkle breadcrumbs over broccoli mixture and drizzle melted butter on top of breadcrumbs. Bake in oven for 30 minutes until slightly crispy and golden brown.

Buttered Corn 🥄 *(4-6 servings)*

16 oz. frozen corn, thawed
2 tbsp. unsalted butter

1 cup water
¼ tsp. sea salt

Combine corn, butter, and water in a medium size sauce pan on medium heat. Cover and cook for about 10 minutes, stirring occasionally. When hot, stir in salt and serve.

Buttered Rice 🥄 *(4-6 servings)*

½ cup unsalted butter
1 cup white rice

2 cups gluten-free chicken broth
salt and pepper, to taste

Melt butter in a pan on medium heat. Stir in rice and cook for 1 minute, then add chicken broth and stir again. Cover and cook for 12-15 minutes, stirring occasionally. Season with salt and pepper before serving.

Candied Sweet Potatoes 🥄🥄 *(10-12 servings)*

6 large sweet potatoes
½ cup unsalted butter, melted
1 ½ cups light brown sugar
1 tbsp. vanilla

1 tsp. ground cinnamon
1 tsp. ground nutmeg
½ tsp. salt

Preheat oven to 375 degrees. Peel and slice sweet potatoes into ¼ inch slices. Grease a 9x13 inch baking dish with cooking spray, layer potato slices in dish. In a medium size mixing bowl, combine butter, sugar, vanilla, cinnamon, nutmeg, and salt. Stir together until well combined, then spread on top of sweet potatoes. Cover with aluminum foil, bake for about 1 hour or until potatoes are fork tender.

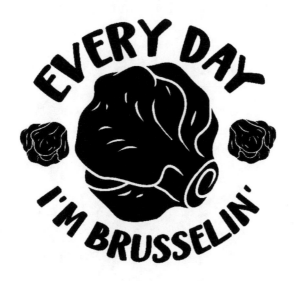

Cheese Ravioli with Roasted Red Peppers and Baby Spinach ♙ (4-6 servings)

¼ cup unsalted butter
¼ cup gluten-free all-purpose flour (no XG)
2 cups half and half
½ cup grated parmesan cheese
1 tsp. Italian seasoning

½ cup diced roasted red bell peppers
½ teaspoon sea salt
2 cups baby spinach leaves
24 oz. gluten-free cheese ravioli

Melt butter in a pot on medium heat, whisk in flour and cook for 1 minute. Slowly pour in half and half, whisking to break up clumps of flour. Continue to cook on medium heat for about 10 minutes, whisking occasionally to make sure clumps don't form in the sauce. When sauce has thickened, turn off heat and parmesan, Italian seasoning, bell peppers, and salt, stirring until cheese has melted. Add spinach and stir just until wilted. Cook ravioli according to package directions, drain. Add pasta to sauce and serve warm.

Cheesy Potato Casserole ♙ (6-8 servings)

½ cup unsalted butter
½ cup gluten-free all-purpose flour (no XG)
4 cups whole milk

½ tablespoon salt
24 oz. grated sharp cheddar cheese
32 oz. frozen diced potatoes, thawed

Preheat oven to 375 degrees. Melt butter in a pot at medium heat, whisk in flour and cook for 1 minute. Slowly pour in milk, whisking to break up clumps of flour. Continue to cook on medium heat for about 10 minutes, whisking occasionally to make sure clumps don't form in the sauce. When sauce has thickened, turn off heat and add salt and 1 lb. cheddar cheese, stirring until cheese has melted. Add potatoes, stir well. Spoon into greased 9x13 inch baking dish, top with remaining cheddar. Place in oven to bake for 55-65 minutes, or until hot and potatoes are tender.

♙ **Pro-Tip:** it is extremely important for the potatoes to be completely thawed, otherwise you'll wait what feels like 3 years for them to become tender during the cooking process.

Coconut Lime Rice ♙ (4-6 servings)

2 tbsp. coconut oil
1 cup white rice
¼ cup frozen grated coconut, thawed
1 lime, zested and juiced

1 cup coconut milk
1 cup chicken broth
¼ tsp. salt
¼ tsp. pepper

Heat coconut oil in a skillet over medium heat. Add rice and coconut, stir and cook for about 2-3 minutes. Add lime juice, zest, coconut milk, and chicken broth. Bring to a gentle boil, then reduce heat, cover and cook for about 15 minutes, until rice is tender. Add salt and pepper, fluff with a fork and serve warm.

Collard Greens (6-8 servings)

¼ cup unsalted butter
1 large onion, chopped
2 cloves garlic, minced
1 lb. fresh collard greens, sliced
3 cups chicken or vegetable broth
½ cup real bacon bits
1 tsp. salt
1 tsp. granulated sugar

Heat butter in a large pot on medium heat, add onion and cook until tender. Add garlic, stir and cook just until fragrant. Add collard greens, cook until they start to wilt. Pour in chicken broth, add bacon bits, salt, and sugar. Reduce heat to low, cover, and cook until greens are tender, about 45 minutes. Serve warm.

Cooked Sweet Carrots (4-6 servings)

16 oz. bag baby carrots
½ cup water
2 tbsp. butter
2 tbsp. light brown sugar
¼ tsp. salt

In a pan on medium heat, combine carrots, water, butter, and brown sugar. Bring to a boil and stir together well. Cover and reduce heat, cook for about 6-8 minutes. Return heat to high, stir occasionally and continue to cook for another 6 minutes, until carrots are tender. Sprinkle with salt and serve warm.

Corn and Rice Cakes (6-8 servings)

1 cup cooked white rice
½ cup gluten-free breadcrumbs
½ cup grated cheddar cheese
¾ cup frozen corn, thawed
½ tsp. salt
1 tbsp. Italian seasoning
2 large eggs, beaten
¼ cup olive oil

In a medium size mixing bowl, combine rice, breadcrumbs, cheese, corn, salt, and Italian seasoning. Toss together well. Add eggs and mix well. Measure 1/3 cup of rice mixture and shape into a patty. Place on a parchment paper lined baking sheet and repeat process until all of rice mixture is used. Heat oil in a large skillet over medium heat. Add patties in a single layer and cook on each side until golden brown, about 2-3 minutes on each side. Serve warm.

Country Vegetables *(4-6 servings)*

2 tbsp. butter
¼ cup chicken or vegetable broth
12 oz. frozen mixed vegetables

1 tsp. granulated sugar
¼ tsp. salt
¼ tsp. black pepper

Melt butter in medium saucepan or skillet. Add broth and stir, then add vegetables. Cover and cook on medium heat for about 10-12 minutes, or until vegetables are tender. Sprinkle sugar, salt, and pepper on vegetables and stir. Serve warm.

Pro-Tip: the mixed vegetables used in this recipe is the medley with corn, peas, carrots, and green beans. You can mix it up using different medleys for a variety, but this is the blend used here.

Creamed Corn *(6-8 servings)*

2 tbsp. butter
1 tbsp. gluten-free all-purpose flour (no XG)
1 lb. frozen corn, thawed
1 cup half and half

½ tsp. salt
1 tsp. granulated sugar
¼ tsp. black pepper
¼ cup grated parmesan cheese

In a skillet over medium heat, melt butter. Whisk in flour with butter and cook for about one minute. Add corn and half and half to skillet, cook stirring over medium heat until the mixture is thickened, and corn is cooked through (about 10 minutes). Add salt, sugar, and pepper to corn, stir. Remove from heat and stir in parmesan cheese until melted, serve hot.

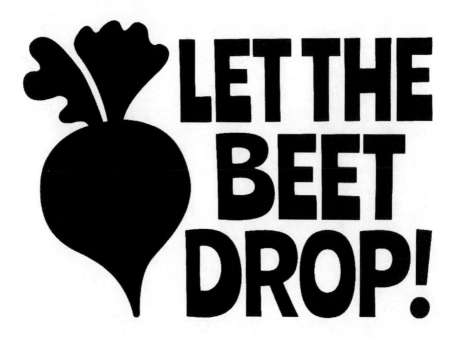

Creamy Mashed Potatoes ∤ (4-6 servings)

24 oz. bag frozen "steam 'n mash" potatoes
½ cup unsalted butter
½ cup milk

¼ tsp. salt
¼ tsp. black pepper

Cook potatoes according to package directions in the microwave. While potatoes are cooking, heat the butter and milk in a small saucepan on medium heat. When mixture is melted and hot, turn to low heat to keep hot. When potatoes are done cooking, cut open the bag and dump potatoes into a medium size mixing bowl. Mash well with a potato masher. Add melted butter and milk, beat at medium speed with electric mixer until well-blended. Add salt and pepper. Continue mixing with electric mixer until creamy. Serve warm.

Eggplant Parmesan ⁉ (4-6 servings)

1 large eggplant
24 oz. spaghetti sauce
1 cup grated parmesan cheese, divided

2 cups grated mozzarella cheese
½ cup gluten-free breadcrumbs
2 tbsp. olive oil

Preheat oven to 375 degrees. Peel and cut eggplant into ¼ inch slices. Preheat oven to 375 degrees. Coat 8x8 inch baking dish with cooking spray. Pour ½ cup sauce in bottom of dish, then place half of eggplant slices over sauce. Spread ½ cup sauce over eggplant slices, sprinkle ½ cup grated Parmesan cheese and 1 cup mozzarella cheese on top. Layer remaining eggplant slices on top, followed by remaining sauce, Parmesan, and mozzarella. Sprinkle breadcrumbs over cheese, drizzle olive oil over breadcrumbs. Bake in oven for 45-50 minutes. Let rest for 10 minutes after baking. Serve hot over pasta.

Fried Green Tomatoes ⁉ (4-6 servings)

3 medium, firm green tomatoes
Salt
1 cup gluten-free all-purpose flour
1 tbsp. Cajun seasoning
½ cup buttermilk

1 large egg
1/3 cup fine gluten-free cornmeal
½ cup gluten-free breadcrumbs
½ cup vegetable oil, for frying

Cut unpeeled tomatoes into ½ inch slices, sprinkling each one with salt and discarding ends. Let sit for five minutes. In one bowl, combine flour and Cajun seasoning. In another bowl, whisk together buttermilk and egg. In a third bowl, combine cornmeal and breadcrumbs. Heat oil in a skillet on medium heat, dip the tomato slices first in the flour mixture, followed by buttermilk mixture, then breadcrumb mix. Fry half tomato slices at a time, 3-5 minutes per side or until golden brown. Set on paper towels to drain, serve warm with Remoulade Sauce (p. 90).

Fried Rice ☘ *(6-8 servings)*

2 tbsp. sesame oil
1 small white onion, diced
2 eggs, beaten

1 cup frozen peas and carrots, thawed
2-3 tbsp. gluten-free soy sauce
3 cups cooked white rice*

Heat a large skillet or wok on medium heat and add sesame oil. Add onion, sauté until tender. Slide the onion to the side, add eggs and scramble using a spatula. When done cooking, add peas and carrots, stir together. Add soy sauce and rice to mixture, stir together until hot and ready to serve.

☘ **Pro-Tip:** make rice the day before and store in the refrigerator until ready to use. This keeps it from getting mushy and is a crucial step!

Green Bean Casserole ☘ *(6-8 servings)*

2 lbs. frozen cut green beans, thawed
10.5 oz. gluten-free cream of mushroom soup
6 oz. can gluten-free French-fried onions

½ cup grated parmesan
½ cup real bacon bits

Preheat oven to 350 degrees. Combine green beans, parmesan, and soup in a medium size mixing bowl, stir together before spreading into a greased 9x13 inch baking dish. Sprinkle bacon bits on top, followed by fried onions. Bake in oven for 35-45 minutes, serve warm.

Green Beans ☘ *(4-6 servings)*

2 tbsp. butter
1 tbsp. olive oil
1 cup water

12 oz. fresh green beans
¼ tsp. salt
¼ tsp. black pepper

Heat butter and olive oil in skillet on medium heat on stove. When butter has melted, add water and green beans, stir. Cover and cook for about 15 minutes, stirring occasionally. When green beans are cooked through and tender, sprinkle salt and pepper, stir to combine. Serve warm.

Grilled Portabello Mushrooms (4 servings)

2 tbsp. balsamic vinegar
2 tbsp. olive oil
1 tbsp. lemon juice

2 cloves garlic, minced
½ tsp. sea salt
4 large portobello mushrooms

Combine balsamic vinegar, olive oil, lemon juice, garlic, and salt in a small mixing bowl and whisk together well. Using a damp paper towel, wipe the mushrooms clean and pull or cut off the stems. Using a spoon, scrape out the gills. Use a pastry brush to coat the gill side with about 1/3 of marinade. Heat a grill pan or outdoor grill on medium heat and grease well. Place each mushroom (gill side down) on grill and cook until browned and tender, about 4-5 minutes. Brush another 1/3 of marinade on tops of mushrooms before flipping over. Continue grilling until brown and tender, another 2-3 minutes. Transfer to a plate and brush with remaining marinade, serve warm.

Grilled Vegetable Skewers (8-12 servings)

3 medium zucchini
3 medium yellow squash
4 red bell peppers
3 medium red onions
12 oz. mushrooms (button or cremini)

½ cup olive oil, divided
5 cloves garlic, minced
salt and pepper to taste
balsamic vinegar

Soak 8-12 wooden skewers in water for 20-30 minutes. Slice zucchini and squash into 1-inch rounds, discarding ends. Seed and cut bell peppers into 1-inch pieces. Peel and slice each onion in half, then cut each half into thirds. Using a damp paper towel, wipe off mushrooms and remove stems. In a small mixing bowl, combine ¼ cup olive oil and garlic, stir together and set aside. Preheat grill to medium/high heat. Skewer the vegetables by alternating each one, then brush with a light layer of remaining olive oil. Add skewers to grill when it's hot, cook for 5-8 minutes on each side until veggies are softening and browning around the edges. Remove from heat, brush with olive oil mixture, sprinkle with salt and pepper, and drizzle with balsamic vinegar if desired.

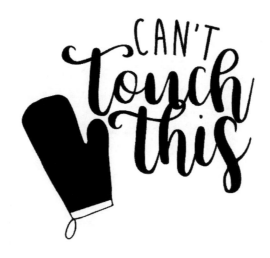

Hashbrown Casserole 👫 *(8-10 servings)*

16 oz. sour cream
½ teaspoon salt
½ cup butter, melted
10.5 oz. can gluten-free cream of chicken soup

32 oz. frozen shredded potatoes, thawed
½ cup diced onion
2 cups grated sharp cheddar cheese
½ cup real bacon bits

Preheat oven to 350 degrees. In a large mixing bowl, whisk together sour cream, salt, butter, and soup. Add hashbrowns, onion, and 1 ½ cups cheese. Stir together well and spoon into a greased 9x13 inch baking dish. Sprinkle remaining cheese and bacon bits on top. Bake for 50-60 minutes, or until hot and bubbly. Serve warm.

Loaded Mashed Potatoes 👫 *(6-8 servings)*

3 medium/large russet potatoes
½ cup unsalted butter
½ cup half and half
¼ cup hot water
0.4 oz. package ranch dressing

½ cup sour cream
1-2 tsp. salt
1 cup grated sharp cheddar cheese
½ cup real bacon bits
2 green onions, sliced

Preheat oven to 350 degrees, peel and cut potatoes into 2-inch cubes. Put potatoes in a large pot with salted water, bring to a boil and cook until tender, about 25 minutes. While potatoes are cooking, heat the butter and half and half in a small saucepan on medium heat. When mixture is melted and hot, turn to low heat. When potatoes are done cooking, dump into a large mixing bowl, mash well with a potato masher. Add melted butter, hot water, and half and half, beat at medium speed with electric mixer until well-blended. Add ranch dressing mix, sour cream, and salt. Continue mixing with electric mixer until creamy. Spoon mashed potatoes into a greased 9x13 inch baking dish, spread into an even layer. Sprinkle cheddar cheese and bacon bits on top. Bake for 35-45 minutes, until hot and cheese is melted. Garnish with green onions.

Mexican Rice 👤 *(6-8 servings)*

¼ cup olive oil
1 cup uncooked long grain rice
1 tsp. garlic salt

½ tsp. ground cumin
2 cups chicken or vegetable broth
½ cup tomato sauce

In a large saucepan over medium heat, add oil and rice. Cook, stirring constantly, until puffed and golden, about 2-3 minutes. Add garlic salt and cumin, stir. Add chicken broth and bring to a boil. Reduce heat to low/medium, cover, and simmer for about 20 minutes, stirring occasionally until rice is tender. Stir in tomato sauce just before serving and serve hot.

Mushroom Marsala 🍴 *(4-6 servings)*

¼ cup unsalted butter
1 lb. mushrooms, sliced
8 oz. gluten-free penne pasta
1 tbsp. minced garlic

2/3 cup marsala cooking wine
1 1/3 cup vegetable broth, divided
1 tbsp. cornstarch
½ cup heavy cream

Melt butter in skillet on medium heat. Add mushrooms and cook until tender (about 8-10 minutes), stirring occasionally. While mushrooms are cooking, boil the pasta in a separate pot according to the package directions, drain, and set them aside. Add garlic to mushrooms, stir, and continue to cook for another minute. Slowly stir in cooking wine, followed by 1 cup vegetable broth. Combine the remaining vegetable broth and cornstarch in a cup, whisk together well until cornstarch has dissolved completely. Slowly stir in with other ingredients. Sauce will take a couple minutes to thicken. Add heavy cream to sauce; stir to combine. Add drained pasta. Serve warm.

Mushroom Risotto 🍴 *(6-8 servings)*

3 tablespoons olive oil, divided
1 lb. button or cremini mushrooms, sliced
2 cloves garlic, minced
½ small onion, diced
1 ½ cups arborio rice
½ cup dry white wine

4 cups chicken or vegetable broth
½ tsp. salt
¼ tsp. pepper
1 tbsp. finely chopped chives
2 tbsp. unsalted butter
¼ cup grated parmesan cheese

Heat 2 tablespoons olive oil in a large saucepan over medium heat. Stir in mushrooms, cook until soft. Add garlic and cook for another minute, until fragrant. Remove mushrooms and liquid to a bowl, set aside. Add remaining tablespoon olive oil to skillet, add onions and stir. Cook until onions are slightly tender, add rice and stir again, cooking for about 2 minutes. When the rice has taken on a pale, golden color, add wine and stir constantly until wine is fully absorbed. Add ½ cup chicken broth to rice, stir until absorbed. Continue adding broth ½ cup at a time, stirring continuously until the liquid is absorbed and rice is al dente, about 15-20 minutes. Add salt and pepper, stir. Remove from heat, stir in mushrooms with liquid, butter, chives, and parmesan. Stir until butter and parmesan has melted, serve warm.

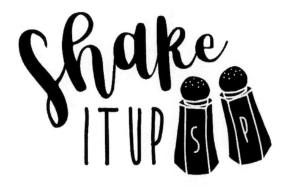

Our Favorite Broccoli ℹ *(4-6 servings)*

2 tbsp. butter
½ cup water

12 oz. bag fresh broccoli florets
¼ teaspoon salt

Place butter in a skillet on medium heat. Once butter is melted, add water and stir. Add broccoli and stir again, cover. Continue to cook on medium heat, stirring occasionally, for about 15 minutes (until broccoli is tender and slightly soft). Sprinkle salt on broccoli, stir again and serve.

Oven Baked Fries ℹ *(4-6 servings)*

¼ cup olive oil, divided
5-6 medium russet potatoes, peeled

1 tsp. seasoned salt

Preheat oven to 400 degrees. Rub 1 tablespoon olive oil into bottom of baking pan, place pan in oven while preheating. Peel and cut potatoes into ½ inch slices, combine in a medium size mixing bowl with olive oil and seasoned salt. Remove baking sheet from oven when heated, spread potatoes onto sheet, bake for about 45-55 minutes or until potatoes are golden brown and tender.

When my daughter is asked what her favorite French Fries are, this is her response. It makes me chuckle but is also a relief that she's not claiming to love any and all fries at other fast-food restaurants. I'll take it.

Pan-Fried Eggplant ℹ *(4-6 servings)*

olive oil, for frying
1 large eggplant
½ cup gluten-free all-purpose flour

1 egg + 1 tbsp. water
½ cup gluten-free breadcrumbs
24 oz. spaghetti sauce

Pour enough olive oil in a skillet to be about ½ inch deep and turn heat to medium. Trim the ends of eggplant; peel and cut into ½ inch round slices. Set up 3 bowls: one for flour, one for egg and water, and one for breadcrumbs. Beat egg and water together. When oil is hot, dredge one piece of eggplant in flour on both sides, then dip in egg on both sides, and coat both sides in breadcrumbs. Place in hot oil to start frying. Fry on each side for 2-3 minutes, until a light golden brown. When each piece is done cooking, lay on a plate lined with a paper towel. Heat marinara in small saucepan on stove. When all pieces are done cooking, arrange on plates and top with marinara. Serve warm.

Penne alla Vodka ♔ (6-8 servings)

1 medium onion, diced
2 tablespoons olive oil
4 garlic cloves, minced
1 teaspoon dried Italian seasoning
6 oz. tomato paste

¼ cup vodka
½ cup prepared pesto
salt and pepper to taste
1 ½ cups heavy cream
1 lb. gluten-free penne pasta

Cook onion with coconut oil in a skillet pan on medium heat until tender, add garlic and Italian seasoning, stir. Add tomato paste and vodka, stir again and continue cooking. Stir in pesto, salt, pepper, and heavy cream until well-combined. While sauce is cooking, cook pasta according to package directions, drain. Sauce will be thick; you can add hot pasta water to thin out sauce to your desired consistency. Add pasta to sauce and serve.

Potato Cakes ♔ (6-8 servings)

24 oz. bag frozen "steam 'n mash" potatoes
1 cup gluten-free all-purpose flour
1 egg, beaten

½ tsp. pepper
½ tsp. salt
1 tsp. onion powder
½ vegetable oil, for frying

Cook potatoes according to package directions in microwave, then mash well with a potato masher in a medium size mixing bowl. Add flour, egg, pepper, salt, and onion powder. Beat with electric mixer until well combined. Using a medium size cookie scoop, scoop mixture into hot oil and lightly press down with a flat spatula. Cook until golden brown, about 4-5 minutes on each side. Drain on paper towels and serve warm.

Potato Gnocchi ♔ (4-6 servings)

24 oz. bag frozen "steam 'n mash" potatoes
1 cup gluten-free all-purpose flour

2 large egg yolks
6 tbsp. butter

Prepare potatoes according to package directions, dump into a medium size mixing bowl and thoroughly mash *very* well with a potato masher. Let cool for 10 minutes. Add flour, egg yolks, and salt, gently fold just until combined and dough comes together. Do not knead or overwork. Separate into four balls and dust a piece of parchment paper with more flour. Roll one piece into a ¾ inch thick rope, about 9 inches long. Cut into ¾ inch gnocchi pieces and roll each piece against the tines of a fork to make ridges. Transfer to prepared baking sheet and repeat process with other 3 dough balls. Bring a large pot of salted water to a rolling boil. Add half of gnocchi to boiling water and gently stir once. Cook for about 2 minutes, then one more minute and reduce heat as necessary to maintain gentle boil. Melt 3 tbsp. butter in a large skillet over medium/high heat. Use a slotted spoon to transfer cooked gnocchi to skillet. Sauté for about 1 minute, adding hot gnocchi water as needed. Remove from skillet, repeat process with remaining gnocchi. season with salt and pepper and serve.

Potatoes au Gratin 🍴 *(4-6 servings)*

3 lbs. russet potatoes
salt and pepper
2 tbsp. butter

2 cups heavy cream
½ cup grated gruyere cheese

Preheat oven to 400 degrees. Peel and slice potatoes into ¼ inch slices. Layer potatoes in a 8x8 inch baking dish and sprinkle with salt and pepper. Cut butter into little chunks and space out on top of potatoes. Pour heavy cream on top, cover dish with aluminum foil and bake in oven for about 60-70 minutes, or until potatoes are fork tender. Remove baking dish from oven and pull off foil, sprinkle cheese on top and return to oven for another 10 minutes for cheese to melt. Remove from oven and let sit for 5 minutes before serving.

Pureed Cauliflower 🍴 *(4 servings)*

1 cup chicken broth or water
1 head cauliflower

¼ cup unsalted butter
¼ teaspoon salt

Bring chicken broth or water to a boil in a pot. Cut cauliflower into 1 inch pieces and add to boiling liquid, cover and reduce heat to low for 20 minutes or until cauliflower is very tender. Use slotted spoon to transfer cauliflower to a food processor or blender, add 2-4 tablespoons hot liquid from pot, butter, and salt. Puree until smooth, add salt as needed.

Quinoa Ratatouille 🍴 *(6-8 servings)*

1 cup uncooked quinoa
1 tbsp. olive oil
½ medium onion, diced
2 cloves garlic, minced
14 oz. can diced tomatoes
1 tbsp. Italian seasoning
1 tsp. salt

½ tsp. pepper
1 large eggplant, cubed
1 green bell pepper, seeded and chopped
1 red bell pepper, seeded and chopped
2 medium zucchini, cubed
½ cup grated parmesan
1 cup grated mozzarella cheese

Preheat oven to 375 degrees. Cook quinoa according to package directions (make sure to rinse quinoa before cooking, this process removes the bitterness). Heat olive oil in large nonstick skillet over medium heat, add onion and sauté for 5 minutes, or until softened. Stir in garlic, diced tomatoes, Italian seasoning, salt, and pepper. Continue to cook for another 1-2 minutes, remove from heat. Place remaining chopped vegetables in bottom of a greased 9x13 inch baking dish. Spoon onion and tomato mixture evenly on top of vegetables. Sprinkle with parmesan cheese, spread cooked quinoa on top, followed by mozzarella. Cover with foil and bake for 40-45 minutes. Remove foil and continue baking for another 5 minutes before serving.

Ratatouille (4-6 servings)

6 tbsp. olive oil, divided
1 large eggplant, cubed
1 ½ tsp. salt, divided
2 medium zucchini, cubed
1 medium onion, diced
1 green bell pepper, seeded and chopped

1 red bell pepper, seeded and chopped
3 cloves garlic, minced
14 oz. can diced tomatoes, drained
½ tsp. pepper
2 tsp. chopped fresh thyme
3 tbsp. chopped fresh basil

Heat 3 tablespoons of oil in large nonstick pan on medium heat. Add eggplant and season with ¼ teaspoon salt, cook until soft and starting to brown, about 10-12 minutes. Transfer to a bowl and set aside. Add another tablespoon oil to pan, add zucchini and cook until tender, about 3-4 minutes. Season with ¼ teaspoon salt and remove from pan to set aside. Add the last 2 tablespoons oil to pan and add onion and bell peppers. Cook for about 5 minutes, stirring frequently. Add garlic and cook for another 2-3 minutes. Add tomatoes, pepper, and remaining salt, then add eggplant and cook for about 10 minutes or until eggplant is soft. Add zucchini and cook for another minute, sprinkle with thyme and basil when ready to serve.

This is a dish that can be made in a couple of different ways. This recipe is made the way I learned how to make it in culinary school, with the vegetables diced into cubes and sauteed together rather than sliced and arranged in a baking dish. Either way, it contains roughly the same ingredients and is packed with all kinds of healthy goodness.

Rice Pilaf (4-6 servings)

½ cup gluten-free spaghetti
1 cup white rice
1 tsp. onion powder
½ tsp. garlic powder
½ tsp. dried parsley

½ tsp. dried thyme
¼ tsp. salt
2 tbsp. unsalted butter
3 cups chicken broth

Break spaghetti into ½ inch pieces and place in a small mixing bowl. Add rice, onion powder, garlic powder, parsley, thyme, and salt, toss together to combine. Melt butter in a skillet pan on medium heat. Add rice mixture and stir, cook until golden. Slowly add chicken broth and stir. Cover and reduce heat to low/medium, stir occasionally and cook for 15-20 minutes or until liquid has been absorbed. Remove from heat and stir, let sit for 2 minutes before serving.

Roasted Asparagus ⚭ *(4-6 servings)*

2 bunches medium asparagus spears
¼ cup olive oil
2 cloves garlic, minced

½ tsp. salt
¼ tsp. black pepper
2 tbsp. lemon juice

Preheat oven to 425 degrees. Trim asparagus spears to remove the thickest part of the ends. In a medium size mixing bowl, combine asparagus, olive oil, and garlic, toss to combine. Arrange evenly in a greased 9x13 inch baking dish. Bake in oven until tender, about 12-15 minutes. Sprinkle with salt and pepper, drizzle with lemon juice just before serving.

Roasted Brussel Sprouts ⚭ *(4-6 servings)*

1 ½ lbs. brussels sprouts
3 tbsp. olive oil
1 tbsp. balsamic vinegar

1 tbsp. maple syrup
½ tsp. salt
½ tsp. pepper

Preheat oven to 425 degrees, line a baking sheet with aluminum foil and set aside. Cut off ends and half each brussel sprout, peel off 1-2 outside layers. In a medium size mixing bowl, combine sprouts, olive oil, balsamic vinegar and maple syrup. Toss together to combine well before spreading onto baking sheet. Place in oven to bake for about 20 minutes or until tender and golden brown, stirring once during baking time. Remove pan from oven, sprinkle with salt and pepper and serve.

Roasted Cauliflower ⚭ *(4-6 servings)*

1 head cauliflower
2 tbsp. olive oil
2 tbsp. butter, melted

¼ tsp. paprika
¼ tsp. salt

Preheat oven to 425 degrees, line a baking sheet with aluminum foil and set aside. Cut the cauliflower into ½ inch pieces, making sure they are all close in size to ensure even baking. In a medium size mixing bowl, combine cauliflower, olive oil, melted butter, and paprika. Toss together well before spreading onto baking sheet. Place baking sheet in oven and roast for 15-20 minutes, or until cauliflower reaches desired consistency. Sprinkle with salt and serve warm.

Roasted Chipotle & Cinnamon Sweet Potatoes *(4-6 servings)*

3 medium size sweet potatoes
3 tbsp. olive oil
½ tsp. ground chipotle pepper

1 tsp. cinnamon
½ tsp. salt

Preheat oven to 375 degrees. In a medium size mixing bowl, combine sweet potatoes, olive oil, chipotle pepper, and cinnamon. Toss together until potatoes are evenly coated. Grease a 9x13 inch baking dish with cooking spray, pour potatoes into baking dish and spread into an even layer. Bake for 45-55 minutes, until potatoes are crispy and tender. Remove from oven, sprinkle salt and toss together in pan before serving.

Roasted Fingerling Potatoes *(4-6 servings)*

1 ½ lbs. fingerling potatoes
2 tbsp. butter, melted
2 tbsp. olive oil

3 cloves garlic, minced
1 tbsp. Italian seasoning
½ tsp. salt

Preheat oven to 425 degrees, line a baking sheet with aluminum foil and set aside. Slice fingerling potatoes in half lengthwise. In a medium size mixing bowl, combine potatoes, butter, olive oil, garlic, and Italian seasoning, toss together to combine well before spreading onto baking sheet. Place baking sheet in oven and bake for 25-30 minutes, or until golden brown and crispy. Sprinkle with salt and serve.

Roasted Red Potatoes *(4-6 servings)*

1 lb. small red potatoes
¼ cup olive oil

¼ tsp. salt
¼ tsp. pepper

Preheat oven to 400 degrees. Cut potatoes into wedges (about 4-6 pieces per potato), and place in a small mixing bowl. Pour olive oil over potatoes; stir together so all potatoes are coated evenly with oil. Coat a 9x13 inch baking dish with cooking spray and spoon potatoes into dish. Place in oven and bake for about 1 hour, stirring potatoes after 30 minutes. Potatoes will be a golden brown when they are done cooking. Remove from oven, sprinkle with desired salt and pepper, and serve warm.

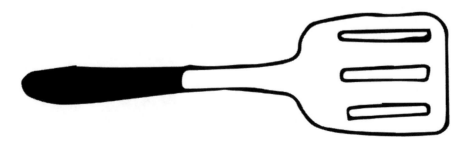

Roasted Sweet Potatoes & Brussels 🍴 *(4-6 servings)*

2 large sweet potatoes
1 lb. brussel sprouts
2 tbsp. olive oil
1 tbsp. maple syrup

2 cloves garlic, minced
1 tsp. Italian seasoning
1 tsp. salt

Preheat oven to 400 degrees. Peel sweet potato and cut off each end, creating a flat side. Cut into bite size pieces (about ½ inch each cubed) and toss into a medium size mixing bowl. Cut off ends and half each brussel sprout, peel off 1-2 outside layers. Toss into bowl with sweet potatoes. In a small bowl, combine olive oil, maple syrup, garlic, and Italian seasoning, whisk together. Pour over vegetables in bowl and lightly toss, making sure all vegetables are coated with the oil. Spray a 9x13 inch baking dish with cooking spray, evenly spread vegetables into one layer. Sprinkle with salt. Bake for 40-45 minutes, until sweet potatoes are tender.

Simple Slaw 🍴 *(4-6 servings)*

1 bag angel hair coleslaw
2/3 cup mayonnaise

½ teaspoon black pepper

In a medium bowl, stir together all ingredients until well combined. Serve immediately or store in refrigerator in airtight container until ready to serve. Store in refrigerator for up to 7 days.

Slow Cooker Corn on the Cob 🍴 *(4 servings)*

4 ears frozen corn on the cob
½ cup unsalted butter, softened
¼ teaspoon garlic powder

¼ teaspoon salt
1/8 teaspoon black pepper

Place softened butter in a bowl and mash with fork. Add garlic powder, salt, and pepper; continue to mash and stir until well-blended. Tear 4 pieces of aluminum foil, each piece large enough to cover one ear of corn. Place each ear of corn on a piece of foil, spread about 2 tablespoons of butter mixture on top of each ear. Roll up corn in pieces of foil, twisting the ends to make sure each piece is entirely covered. Lay each one flat in a slow cooker (at least 4-quart size), and pour water in the bottom, until it's a little less than halfway up each ear of corn. Set slow cooker to low setting and cover. Cook on low for 4-5 hours, until corn is tender and ready to eat.

Slow Cooker Lima Beans *(4-6 servings)*

12 oz. chicken or vegetable broth
12 oz. bag frozen lima beans
½ tsp. onion powder

2 tbsp. unsalted butter
¼ tsp. salt
¼ tsp. black pepper

Pour chicken broth in a small (1.5 quart) slow cooker. Add lima beans and onion powder and stir together. Cook on low for 8-10 hours (until beans are soft and tender), stir in butter to melt, add salt and pepper before serving.

Slow Cooker Mac 'n Cheese *(12-14 servings)*

16 oz. gluten-free elbow macaroni
8 oz. block sharp white cheddar cheese
16 oz. block sharp cheddar cheese
1 cup butter
1 tsp. Dijon mustard

1 tsp. salt
½ tsp. black pepper
4 eggs, beaten
2 cans evaporated milk
3 cups whole milk

Cook macaroni noodles according to package directions and drain. While noodles are cooking, grate cheese. Place butter in a microwave safe bowl and melt. When butter is melted, whisk in the mustard, salt and pepper until blended. Reserve 1 cup of cheese to use as topping. Combine all ingredients in slow cooker, sprinkle reserved cheese on top. Cover and cook on low for 3 hours. Turn setting to low and serve hot.

Southwest Corn Casserole *(4-6 servings)*

6 tbsp. butter, melted
2 lbs. frozen corn kernels, thawed
¼ cup gluten-free cornmeal
½ tsp. garlic salt

4 oz. can diced green chiles
2 eggs, beaten
2 cups grated cheddar

Preheat oven to 350 degrees. Pour melted butter into 8x8 inch baking dish. In a medium size mixing bowl, combing remaining ingredients and stir together well before spooning into dish. Bake for 1 hour, until golden brown. Serve warm.

Southwestern Style Veggies ♙ *(4-6 servings)*

2 tbsp. olive oil or butter
2 medium zucchini
1 red bell pepper
1 small onion, diced
1 clove garlic, minced

1 lb. frozen corn, thawed
1 tsp. ground cumin
¼ tsp. salt
¼ tsp. pepper
¼ cup chopped fresh cilantro

Heat oil in a large non-stick skillet on medium heat. Slice zucchini into ¼ inch pieces and discard ends, then seed and dice bell pepper. Set veggies aside. Add onion and cook until tender, then add zucchini, bell peppers and garlic. Continue cooking until tender, add corn, cumin, salt, and pepper, stir and cover. Cook for another five minutes, until hot. Remove from heat, garnish with cilantro and serve.

Spinach Au Gratin ♙ *(4-6 servings)*

1 tbsp. butter
4 oz. cream cheese, softened
¾ cup heavy cream
½ tsp. onion powder
½ tsp. garlic powder

¼ tsp. salt
¼ tsp. pepper
½ cup grated Swiss cheese
¼ cup grated parmesan cheese
20 oz. chopped frozen spinach, thawed

Preheat oven to 400 degrees. Heat a nonstick skillet on medium heat, add butter and cream cheese. Cook until butter and cream cheese start to melt, add heavy cream and stir together well, continue cooking about 2 minutes or until sauce thickens. Stir in onion powder, garlic powder, salt, and pepper. Remove from heat, add Swiss and parmesan cheeses and stir. Squeeze spinach dry, then evenly spread into 8x8 inch baking dish, pour cream mixture on top. Place dish in oven and bake for 15-20 minutes, or until hot. Let sit for 5 minutes before serving.

Squash Casserole ♙ *(6-8 servings)*

4 cups sliced yellow squash
½ cup onion, diced
¼ cup water
1 cup gluten-free breadcrumbs
1 cup grated cheddar cheese

2 eggs, beaten
¾ cup milk
¼ cup butter, melted
1 tsp. salt
¼ tsp. pepper

Preheat oven to 400 degrees. Combine squash, onion, and water in a large skillet on medium heat. Cover and cook until squash is tender. Drain well before transferring to a medium size mixing bowl. In a small mixing bowl, combine the breadcrumbs and cheddar, toss together then add half of mixture into bowl with squash. Mix eggs and milk together before pouring into bowl with squash. Add melted butter, salt, and pepper. Stir together well to combine, spread into 8x8 inch baking dish. Sprinkle remaining breadcrumb mixture on top, bake in oven for about 25 minutes.

Stuffed Bell Peppers (4 servings)

4 large green bell peppers
1 cup diced onion
8 oz. sliced mushrooms

8 oz. garden blend cream cheese spread
½ tsp. salt
3 cups grated cheddar, divided

Preheat oven to 350 degrees. Cut off tops of bell peppers, remove center, and scoop out any seeds. In a medium sized mixing bowl, combine the onion, mushrooms, cream cheese, salt, and 2 cups grated cheddar. Beat with electric mixer at medium speed until well combined. Place each pepper in a baking dish or on a cookie sheet, stuff with veggie mixture, then sprinkle with remaining cheese. Bake for about 45 minutes until peppers are tender and cheese is melted. Serve warm.

Stuffed Portobello Mushrooms (4 servings)

4 portobello mushroom caps
1 tsp. salt, divided
10 oz. frozen chopped spinach, thawed
4 oz. cream cheese, softened

¼ tsp. onion powder
¼ tsp. garlic powder
¼ cup grated parmesan cheese
½ cup grated mozzarella cheese

Preheat oven to 400 degrees. Using a damp paper towel, wipe the mushrooms clean and pull or cut off the stems. Using a spoon, scrape out the gills. Place mushrooms stem side down on baking pan and bake for 10-15 minutes, or until water leaks out. Remove from oven, soak up excess water with paper towels. Place mushrooms cap side down on baking pan and sprinkle with salt. Drain spinach and squeeze out as much water as possible. In a medium size mixing bowl, combine cream cheese, onion powder, garlic powder, and parmesan. Beat with electric mixer until combined, then spoon into each mushroom cap and top with mozzarella cheese. Return to oven and bake for another 10-15 minutes, until hot and cheese is melted.

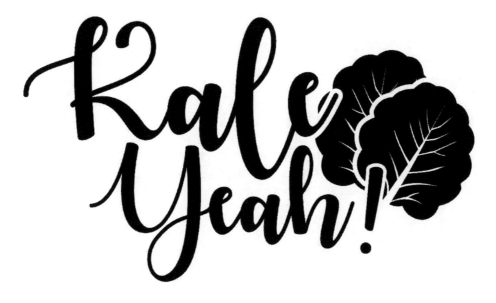

Stuffing (8-10 servings)

24 oz. loaf gluten-free white bread
¾ cup butter
1 medium yellow onion, diced
4 stalks celery, diced
½ tbsp. dried thyme

½ tsp. ground sage
½ tsp. rosemary
1 tsp. salt
½ tsp. black pepper
2-2 ½ cups chicken broth

Let bread slices dry out for at least 1-2 hours before cutting into 1-inch pieces. Preheat oven to 350 degrees. Melt butter in a skillet on medium heat, add onion and celery, cook until tender. Add thyme, sage, rosemary, salt, and pepper, stir together. Add bread cubes and mix until coated evenly before spooning into greased 9x13 inch baking dish. Drizzle broth on top of mixture, bake for 35-45 minutes.

Sweet Potato Casserole (4-6 servings)

40 oz. can yams (sweet potatoes)
¼ cup unsalted butter, melted
½ tsp. cinnamon
1 egg

½ cup light brown sugar
½ cup milk
4-5 jumbo marshmallows

Preheat oven to 350 degrees. Open can of yams and drain liquid out, then pour yams into a medium size mixing bowl. Using a potato masher, mash very well. Add melted butter, cinnamon, egg, light brown sugar, and milk. Using an electric mixer, beat at medium speed for 1-2 minutes until well combined. Spoon into 8x8 inch baking dish. Slice marshmallows in half; place on top of sweet potatoes. Place dish in oven and bake for 30 minutes. Remove from oven and serve warm.

Sweet Potato Fries (4-6 servings)

6 cups peanut oil, for frying
1 teaspoon salt
½ teaspoon paprika

2 lbs. sweet potatoes
1 cup cornstarch
¾ cup club soda

Heat oil in a deep fryer or Dutch oven to 375 degrees. In a small bowl, whisk together the salt and paprika. Peel and cut sweet potatoes into ¼ inch fries. In a medium size mixing bowl, whisk together cornstarch and club soda. Dip potatoes in batter in batches, allow excess to drip off and set on a wire rack. Repeat process with all potatoes. Fry half of potatoes, stirring occasionally until golden brown and crispy, about 6-8 minutes. Transfer to paper towel lined baking pan and sprinkle with half of seasoning. Repeat process with last batch of potatoes, serve warm.

Twice Baked Potatoes 🍴 (4 servings)

5 large baking potatoes
1 tbsp. olive oil
½ tbsp. salt
¼ cup real bacon bits

2 cups grated cheddar, divided
1 cup sour cream
¼ cup butter, softened
2 tbsp. snipped chives

Preheat oven to 400 degrees. Rub potatoes with olive oil, sprinkle with salt and poke holes in potatoes with a fork. Place on baking sheet and bake until fork tender, about 60-70 minutes. Let potatoes rest until cool enough to handle. Peel one potato, discard the skin and place pulp in a mixing bowl. Cut the top quarter lengthwise of each potato, scoop pulp into bowl using a spoon. Leave a ¼ inch layer of pulp on the skin. Return shells to baking sheet. Add bacon, 1 cup cheddar, sour cream, butter, and chives to pulp. Use a potato masher to mash mixture very well. Spoon filling back into each potato shell and sprinkle with remaining cheddar. Bake until cheese is melted, about 15 minutes.

Vegetable Casserole 🍴 (6-8 servings)

10 oz. can gluten-free cream of mushroom soup
¼ tsp. pepper
8 oz. sour cream
2 lbs. frozen mixed veggies, thawed (corn, peas, carrots, green beans)

2 cups grated cheddar cheese
1 cup gluten-free breadcrumbs
½ cup butter, melted

Preheat oven to 350 degrees. Whisk together the soup, pepper, and sour cream in a mixing bowl. Add mixed veggies and cheese, stir together well and spoon into a greased 9x13 inch baking dish. In a small mixing bowl, toss together the breadcrumbs and butter, sprinkle on top of veggies. Bake in oven for 35-45 minutes, serve warm.

Vegetable Paella 🍴 (4-6 servings)

3 tablespoons olive oil
1 medium onion, diced
1 red bell pepper, seeded and diced
5 cloves garlic, minced
½ cup canned diced tomatoes, drained
1 ½ cups arborio rice

1 tsp. dried thyme
1 tsp. ground turmeric
1 ½ tsp. paprika
4 cups vegetable broth
1 tsp. salt
¾ cup frozen peas, thawed

Heat olive oil in a large skillet pan over medium heat. Add onion and bell pepper, cook until softened and lightly browned, about 3-5 minutes. Add garlic and cook for another minute. Add tomatoes, rice, thyme, turmeric, and paprika, stir well. Cook for 1-2 minutes to lightly toast the rice and let the flavors blend together. Slowly pour in vegetable broth and add salt. Bring to a boil, then cover and reduce heat to a medium/low heat and simmer for 15-20 minutes. Add peas and stir before serving.

Vegetable Risotto ♒ (4-6 servings)

2 tablespoons olive oil
1 medium onion, diced
1 red bell pepper, seeded and diced
1 bunch asparagus
6 cups vegetable broth, divided

1 ½ cups arborio rice
½ cup dry white wine
¾ tsp. salt
¼ cup freshly grated parmesan
2 tbsp. unsalted butter

Heat olive oil in a large skillet pan over medium heat. Add onion and bell pepper, cook until softened and lightly browned, about 3-5 minutes. Cut off thick ends of asparagus, then cut the rest into 1-inch pieces. In a saucepan, combine 1 cup vegetable broth and asparagus, cover and cook on medium/high heat until tender. Use a slotted spoon to remove asparagus from pan and set aside. Add rice to onion mixture and toast for about 1 minute, then add white wine. When wine has soaked into rice, add remaining broth ½ cup at a time, stirring continuously until the liquid is absorbed and rice is al dente, about 15-20 minutes. Remove from heat, stir in salt, parmesan, and butter. Stir until butter and parmesan has melted, serve warm.

Vegetarian Lasagna ♒ (6-8 servings)

20 oz. frozen spinach, thawed
20 oz. frozen chopped broccoli, thawed
15 oz. ricotta cheese
¾ cup grated parmesan cheese

2 (24 oz.) jars spaghetti sauce
1 cup water
12 oven-ready gluten-free lasagna noodles
4 cups grated mozzarella cheese

Preheat oven to 350 degrees. Coat a 9x13 inch baking dish with cooking spray. Squeeze as much liquid as possible out of spinach and broccoli, place in a medium size mixing bowl. Add ricotta cheese and ½ cup grated Parmesan, stir together until well combined. In another mixing bowl, combine spaghetti sauce and water, stir together until smooth. Spread ½ cup spaghetti sauce into bottom of baking dish, followed by 4 pieces of lasagna noodles in even layer to cover sauce. Spread half of veggie/ricotta mixture over layer of noodles, followed by 1 cup of spaghetti sauce. Sprinkle 1 cup grated mozzarella over sauce. Repeat layering. Place last 4 pieces of noodles on top, followed by remaining spaghetti sauce, parmesan, and mozzarella. Cover dish with foil and bake for 45 minutes. Remove foil from top and continue baking for another 10 minutes. Remove from oven and allow to stand for 10-15 minutes before serving.

Veggie Stir-Fry *(4-6 servings)*

2 tbsp. olive oil
20 oz. bag frozen stir-fry vegetables
¼ cup chicken or vegetable broth

½ tsp. cornstarch
3 tbsp. gluten-free soy sauce
2 tbsp. honey

In a wok or large non-stick skillet pan, heat oil on medium heat. Add vegetables and fry until vegetables are crisp/tender, about 5-7 minutes. In a small bowl, whisk together broth, cornstarch, soy sauce, and honey. Pour over vegetables and stir, continue to cook until sauce has thickened, 3-4 minutes. Serve warm.

White Bean and Spinach Pasta *(4-6 servings)*

8 oz. gluten-free pasta
2 tbsp. olive oil
3 cloves garlic, minced
1 pint cherry or grape tomatoes, cut in half
¼ tsp. pepper

½ tsp. salt
½ tsp. dried basil
15 oz. can cannellini beans
4 oz. baby spinach
¼ cup freshly grated parmesan

Fill a pot with water and bring to a boil, cook pasta according to package directions for al dente. In a nonstick skillet pan, heat olive oil on medium heat. Add garlic and tomatoes, cook until the tomatoes break down and release their juices into the pan. Stir in pepper, salt, and dried basil. Rinse and drain beans before adding to skillet. Add spinach and continue cooking until it starts to wilt, then add cooked pasta and stir. Spoon into serving dishes and sprinkle with grated parmesan.

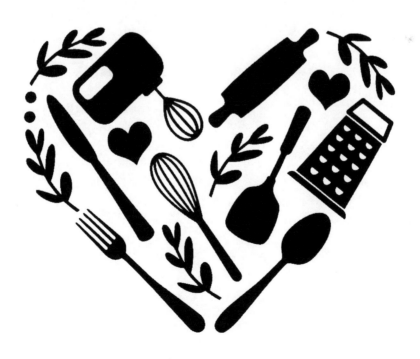

Zucchini Boats ⚱ (4 servings)

2 medium size zucchini
Salt and pepper

½ cup garden blend cream cheese
½ cup grated sharp cheddar cheese

Preheat oven to 375 degrees. Slice zucchini in half, lengthwise. Chop off ends and scoop out center of zucchini with a spoon or melon baller, leaving about a ¼ inch edge around sides and bottom. Sprinkle zucchini with desired salt and pepper, then spread 2 tablespoons cream cheese in each zucchini. Sprinkle 2 tablespoons cheddar on top, place zucchini in baking dish and bake for about 25 minutes, or until zucchini is tender and cheeses are melted. Serve hot.

Zucchini Patties ⚱⚱ (4-6 servings)

2 cups grated zucchini, packed
½ cup gluten-free baking mix
½ cup grated cheddar cheese
1 tsp. onion powder
½ tsp. salt

½ tsp. dried basil
¼ tsp. pepper
2 eggs, beaten
¼ cup olive oil

In a medium size mixing bowl, combine zucchini, baking mix, cheese, onion powder, salt, basil, and pepper, toss to combine. Add eggs and stir together well. Heat olive oil on medium heat in a skillet, drop batter by ¼ cupfuls into hot oil and lightly press down with a spatula. Cook until lightly browned, about 4 minutes on each side. Serve warm with your favorite sauce on the side.

Pro-Tip: be sure to squeeze all the water out of zucchini before mixing, too much moisture will cause them to fall apart during the cooking process.

Zucchini, Squash and Onion Sauté ⚱ (4-6 servings)

2 medium zucchini
2 medium yellow squash
2 tablespoons unsalted butter

1 sweet onion, sliced
¼ teaspoon salt

Slice zucchini and squash into ¼ inch slices. Melt butter in a large skillet on medium heat, add onion, zucchini, and squash. Cover and cook for 10-15 minutes, stirring occasionally. When vegetables are tender, sprinkle with salt and serve warm.

Bakeshop

Almond Flour Biscuits 🍴 *(8-10 servings)*

2 cups almond flour
2 tsp. baking powder
½ tsp. salt

2 eggs, beaten
1/3 cup butter, melted
¼ cup sour cream

Preheat oven to 350 degrees. In a medium size mixing bowl or standing mixer, combine all ingredients and beat at medium speed just until well-combined. Using a cookie scoop, distribute batter onto a silicone lined baking sheet and bake for about 15-16 minutes, until golden and firm. Serve warm, or wrap individually in plastic wrap and store in freezer for up to 6 months.

🍴 **Pro-Tip:** using silicone mats for baking distributes the heat evenly for cookies, biscuits, rolls, etc. so the top and bottom of your baked goods are the same color!

Angel Food Cake 🍴🍴🍴 *(8-10 servings)*

1 ½ cups egg whites
¾ cup gluten-free all-purpose flour
¼ cup cornstarch
¾ cup confectioners sugar
¾ cup granulated sugar

¼ tsp. salt
1 ½ tsp. cream of tartar
1 tbsp. vanilla extract
¼ tsp. almond extract

Sit egg whites aside for at least 30 minutes to allow them to come to room temperature. Preheat oven to 350 degrees. Combine flour, cornstarch, and confectioners sugar in a medium size mixing bowl and whisk together. Pour granulated sugar into a food processor and pulse 5-7 times, just to make it slightly finer than normal and set aside. Place egg whites in another medium size mixing bowl or standing mixer, beat on high speed until they start to foam, then add salt and cream of tartar. Add extracts, continue whipping on high speed. Slowly add the granulated sugar, about 1 tablespoon at a time while they are whipping. Continue to whip until stiff peaks form. Slowly fold in flour mixture 1/3 at a time using a spatula. Be sure to do this slowly and carefully to avoid deflating the egg whites. Spoon into an ungreased 10-inch round tube pan. Bake for 35-40 minutes, until lightly golden. Immediately invert pan onto a cooling rack and cool completely. Run a knife along the edges of the pan and carefully remove cake from the pan. Serve immediately or use in other recipes.

Apple Pie ♙♙ *(6-8 servings)*

1 Pie Crust recipe (p. 222)
6-7 Granny Smith Apples (peeled and cored)
½ tbsp. cinnamon
½ cup butter

3 tbsp. gluten-free all-purpose flour
¼ cup water
1 cup granulated sugar
1 egg + 1 tbsp. water

Preheat oven to 425 degrees. Remove dough disks from refrigerator, let soften slightly (15-20 minutes) before rolling out to ¼ inch thick. Press dough into 9-inch pie plate in the bottom and up the sides. Transfer pie plate to refrigerator while making pie filling. Cut apples into 7 cups of thin slices, place in a large bowl and sprinkle with cinnamon. Melt butter in a medium saucepan over medium heat, whisk in flour and simmer for 1 minute. Whisk in ¼ cup water, sugar, and bring to a boil. Reduce heat and continue to simmer for another 3 minutes, whisking frequently then remove from heat. Pour over apple slices and stir to coat completely, then spoon into pie plate on top of pie crust. Make sure the mound is in the center, so the filling doesn't prevent you from being able to seal the top and bottom pie crusts together. Roll out second pie crust disk to about 11 inches in diameter, then lay on top of pie. Press along the edges of dough with a fork to seal crusts together. Using a sharp knife, cut slits around the middle of the pie. In a small bowl, combine egg and water, beat well then brush the top of the pie crust. Bake at 425 degrees for 15 minutes, then reduce heat to 350 degrees and continue baking for another 45 minutes or until apples are soft and the filling is bubbling through the slits. Rest at room temperature for 1 hour before serving.

❕**Pro-Tip:** place a foil-lined baking sheet under the pie while baking in the oven to catch any filling that may spill over for easy clean up.

Banana Nut Bread ♙♙ *(6-8 servings)*

1 ½ cups gluten-free all-purpose flour
¾ cup light brown sugar
2 tsp. baking powder
1 tsp. baking soda
½ tsp. sea salt

3 very ripe bananas
1 egg
1 tsp. vanilla extract
¼ cup vegetable oil
½ cup chopped pecans

Preheat oven to 350 degrees. In a medium size mixing bowl or standing mixer, combine flour, sugar, baking powder, baking soda, and salt. In a blender, combine bananas, egg, vanilla, oil, and puree until smooth. Pour into mixing bowl with dry ingredients and beat with electric mixer at medium speed until well-combined. Stir in chopped pecans, spoon into greased 9x5 inch loaf pan. Bake for 50-60 minutes, or until a toothpick inserted in center comes out clean. Remove pan from oven and cool on cooling rack for about 20 minutes before turning bread out of pan to cool completely. Slice and serve with Honey Butter (p. 27) for the ultimate experience.

❕**Pro-Tip:** if you're not into nuts, replace pecans with mini chocolate chips.

Boston Crème Trifle *(10-12 servings)*

2 small boxes Jell-O® instant vanilla pudding
3 cups milk
1 recipe Pound Cake (p. 223)

8 oz. frozen whipped topping, thawed
¾ cup heavy cream
1 cup chocolate chips

In a medium size mixing bowl, whisk together pudding mix and milk until well combined. Place in refrigerator to set for at least 5 minutes. Crumble 1/3 of pound cake into the bottom of a trifle dish. Remove pudding from refrigerator, gently stir in whipped topping. Spoon half of pudding mixture on top of pound cake and repeat layering: there will be 3 layers of pound cake, 2 layers of pudding mixture. Place chocolate chips in a small mixing bowl. In a microwave safe dish, heat heavy cream for 45-60 seconds or until it starts to bubble and is hot. Pour hot cream over chocolate chips, whisk together until chocolate is melted and smooth. Spread chocolate over top layer of pound cake. Cover dish with plastic wrap and store in refrigerator for at least 1 hour before serving.

Buckeyes *(50 buckeyes)*

12 tbsp. butter, softened
1 1/3 cups creamy peanut butter

3 cups confectioners sugar
2 (12 oz.) bags chocolate chips

In a medium size mixing bowl, combine butter, peanut butter and confectioners sugar. Using an electric mixer, beat at medium speed for 1-2 minutes until mixture is smooth. Using a mini cookie scoop (about 1 tablespoon), scoop out mixture one by one and place onto parchment paper lined cookie sheet. Place in freezer for about 30 minutes to become firm. Melt chocolate in 20-30 second intervals in microwave in a microwave-safe dish, stirring in between each interval until completely melted and smooth. Using a toothpick or wooden skewer, dip each ball into chocolate, coating ¾ of the ball (leaving top of peanut butter ball exposed). Place on another parchment paper lined cookie sheet, uncoated side up. Let stand until the chocolate hardens. Store in airtight container at room temperature or in refrigerator for up to 1 week.

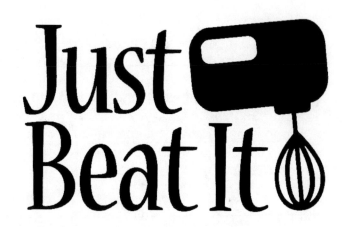

Buckeye Brownies (24 servings)

For the Brownies
2 boxes gluten-free brownie mix
1 cup vegetable oil
4 eggs
¼ cup water

Peanut Butter Layer
12 tbsp. butter, softened
1 2/3 cup creamy peanut butter
2 cups confectioners sugar

Chocolate Ganache
½ cup heavy cream
1 cup chocolate chips

Preheat oven to 350 degrees. Dump brownie mixes into a large mixing bowl. In a small mixing bowl, whisk together the oil, eggs and water. Add wet ingredients to dry ingredients, stir together well. Line a 9x13 inch baking pan with parchment paper hanging over sides, coat with cooking spray. Spoon brownie batter into pan on top of parchment paper and spread into an even layer. Bake brownies for about 45 minutes, or until toothpick inserted in center comes out almost clean. Cool completely on cooling rack. In a medium size mixing bowl, combine butter, peanut butter, and confectioners sugar. Beat with electric mixer until smooth, about 1-2 minutes. Spread peanut butter layer on top of cooled brownies in pan into an even layer. Heat heavy cream in a microwave save dish for 30-45 seconds, or until bubbling. Pour over chocolate chips in a small mixing bowl, whisk together until chocolate chips are melted and smooth. Spread chocolate ganache on top of peanut butter layer into a smooth layer. Place in refrigerator for at least 30 minutes for layers to set. Pull brownies out of pan using the edges of parchment paper and transfer to cutting board before cutting into pieces. Store in airtight container at room temperature for up to 5 days, or wrap individually in plastic wrap and store in freezer for up to 6 months.

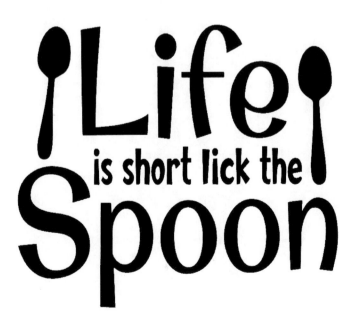

Cheesecake Brownies 🍴 *(24 servings)*

For the Brownies
2 boxes gluten-free brownie mix
1 cup vegetable oil
4 eggs
¼ cup water

Cheesecake Layer
16 oz. cream cheese, softened
2/3 cup granulated sugar
2 eggs
2 tsp. vanilla

Preheat oven to 350 degrees. Line a 9x13 inch baking pan with parchment paper hanging over sides, coat with cooking spray. Dump both bags of brownie mix into a large mixing bowl. Combine oil, 2 eggs, and water in a small mixing bowl and whisk together well. Pour liquid into large mixing bowl with brownie mix and stir together gently with a spatula until well combined. Spoon batter into pan on top of parchment paper and spread into an even layer. In a medium size mixing bowl, combine cream cheese and granulated sugar. Beat with an electric mixer at medium speed until smooth. Add eggs and vanilla, beat again until smooth. Drop in dollops on top of brownie batter, swirl gently with a knife. Place pan in oven and bake for about 50 minutes, until a toothpick inserted in center comes out with just a tiny bit of fudge on tip. Set pan on cooling rack to cool completely. Remove brownies from pan by pulling up sides of parchment paper and transfer to a cutting board. Cut brownies into desired sizes and store in airtight container in refrigerator for 3 days, or wrap individually and store in the freezer for up to 6 months.

Cheesecake Tarts 🍴 *(12 servings)*

12 Gluten-Free Oreo® cookies
2 (8 oz.) cream cheese, softened
1 cup confectioners sugar
1 egg

1 tsp. vanilla
1/3 cup heavy cream
½ cup Gluten-Free Oreo® cookie chunks
Whipped Cream (p. 214)

Preheat oven to 350 degrees. Place cookies in bottom of a muffin pan lined with cupcake liners. Combine cream cheese and confectioners sugar in a medium size mixing bowl and beat with electric mixer at medium speed just until combined. Add egg, vanilla, and heavy cream, mix again just until smooth. Add cookie chunks and stir together before distributing batter evenly on top of cookies in muffin pans. Place pan in oven and bake for 18-20 minutes, remove from oven to cool for 1 hour before transferring to refrigerator for another 2 hours to set. Gently remove from pan, top with whipped cream and serve. Store in refrigerator for up to 5 days, or in freezer for 2 months.

Pro-Tip: For different variations, you can use a different gluten-free cookie as a crust along with different fillings. Examples would be a chocolate chip cookie crust with mini chocolate chips, graham cracker crust with strawberry chunks, etc.

Chocolate Chip Cookies *(2 dozen)*

1 cup oat flour
1 ¾ cups gluten-free all-purpose flour
1 tsp. baking powder
1 tsp. baking soda
1 tsp. salt
1 cup + 2 tbsp. butter, softened

1 cup light brown sugar
1 cup granulated sugar
1 tbsp. molasses
2 eggs
2 tsp. vanilla
12 oz. bag chocolate chips

Preheat oven to 350 degrees. In a small mixing bowl, combine flours, baking powder, baking soda, salt, whisk together and set aside. Combine softened butter and sugars in a medium size mixing bowl and beat at medium speed with electric mixer until light and fluffy. Add molasses, eggs, and vanilla, continue mixing just until combined. Add dry ingredients in two batches, beat in between each to incorporate well. Add chocolate chips and stir. Using a cookie scoop, drop dough on silicone lined cookie sheet and gently press down to form a little hockey puck shaped cookie. Bake for approximately 12 minutes or until lightly golden. Let cookies sit on cookie sheet for another 2-3 minutes before transferring to cooling racks. Store in airtight container at room temperature for up to 3 days, or in freezer for up to 6 months.

Pro-Tip: the combination of oat flour along with the all-purpose flour gives it a perfect balance of consistency compared to traditional cookies.

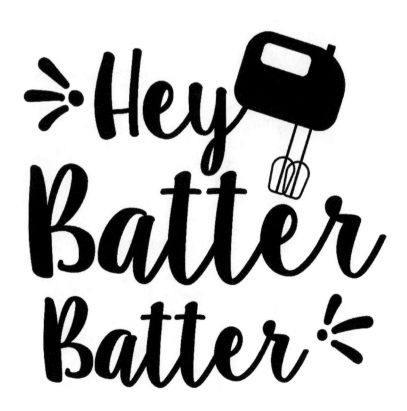

Chocolate Cream Pie 🍴 *(6-8 servings)*

Oreo® Crust
30 gluten-free Oreo® cookies
6 tbsp. butter, melted

Whipped Cream
1 cup heavy cream
1 tbsp. granulated sugar
1 tsp. unflavored gelatin

Chocolate Filling
1/3 cup granulated sugar
2 ½ cups half and half
6 large egg yolks
2 tbsp. cornstarch
6 tbsp. butter
8 oz. good quality chocolate, chopped
½ tbsp. vanilla extract

Preheat oven to 350 degrees. Place cookies in a food processor and process into fine crumbs. Transfer crumbs to a small mixing bowl, toss together with 5 tbsp. melted butter. Press into bottom and up sides of a 9-inch pie plate. Bake in oven for about 10 minutes, until crust is fragrant. Remove from oven and cool completely before filling with chocolate layer.

In a saucepan on medium heat, combine sugar, half and half, whisk well to combine. Bring mixture to a simmer, whisking frequently. Combine the egg yolks and cornstarch in a small mixing bowl and whisk until smooth. Once the cream mixture is simmering, slowly pour in about ½ cup of the hot liquid into the egg yolks and whisk to temper the eggs. Add a little more of the liquid into the egg yolks and whisk again. Then, slowly whisk the egg yolk mixture back into the saucepan. Whisk constantly until the mixture begins to thicken and comes to a very gentle boil (you will see big bubbles break the surface). Remove pan from the heat and pour over the butter, chocolate, and vanilla in a medium size mixing bowl. Stir until completely smooth and chocolate is melted. Pour filling into the cooled pie crust and smooth into an even layer. Place a piece of plastic wrap gently on top and refrigerate until filling is set about 4-6 hours or overnight.

For the Whipped Cream: combine heavy cream and sugar in a standing mixer or mixing bowl, beat at medium/high speed until soft peaks form. Sprinkle in gelatin and continue to beat for another 15-20 seconds. Spoon whipped cream into a pastry bag and pipe on top of chocolate layer with a cake decorating tip, or you can smooth it into an even layer. Garnish with chocolate curls, if desired. Store in refrigerator for up to 5 days.

Pro-Tip: To make this an authentic Chocolate Cream Pie with a sweet pie crust, use one disk from the Pie Crust Recipe (p. 222) and follow as directed:

Let pie dough soften slightly before rolling out to ¼ inch thick. Press dough into a 9-inch pie plate in the bottom and up sides. Poke holes in the dough with a fork, bake crust at 400 degrees for 15-20 minutes or until a light golden brown. Let pie crust cool completely before assembling the chocolate filling and whipped cream topping.

Chocolate Cupcakes ⸕ *(24 cupcakes)*

For the Cupcakes

1 box gluten-free chocolate cake mix*
1 small box Jell-O® instant chocolate pudding mix
¾ cup vegetable oil

½ cup milk
4 eggs
8 oz. sour cream

Preheat oven to 350 degrees. Combine all ingredients in a medium size mixing bowl or standing mixer, beat at medium speed for 1-2 minutes until batter is smooth. Scoop batter into lined muffin pans, place in oven to bake for 21-23 minutes, until a toothpick inserted in center of cupcakes comes out clean. Remove pans from oven, remove cupcakes from pans to cool completely on cooling racks before icing.

*The gluten-free cake mix used in this recipe is King Arthur® brand.
These measurements are based on recipe experiments using this brand. If you use another brand and something comes off wonky, you've been warned. Love you, mean it.

For Chocolate Icing

1 lb. butter, softened
5 cups confectioners sugar
1 cup unsweetened dark cocoa
1 tbsp. vanilla extract
¼ cup milk

For Cookies 'n Cream Icing

1 lb. butter, softened
5 cups confectioners sugar
1 cup gluten-free Oreo® crumbs
1 tbsp. vanilla extract
¼ cup milk

Beat butter at high speed in a medium size mixing bowl or standing mixer for at least 3 minutes, until light and fluffy. Add remaining ingredients and beat slowly to incorporate, then increase speed to high and continue mixing for another 2-3 minutes. Spoon into a pastry bag with cake decorating tip and pipe on top of cupcakes.

For Peanut Butter Icing

1 lb. butter, softened
½ cup peanut butter
5 cups confectioners sugar
1 tbsp. vanilla extract

For Cream Cheese Icing

1 cup butter, softened
8 oz. cream cheese, softened
6 cups confectioners sugar
1 tbsp. vanilla extract

Combine the first two ingredients in a medium size mixing bowl or standing mixer and beat at high speed for at least 3 minutes, until light and fluffy. Add remaining ingredients and beat slowly to incorporate, then increase speed to high and continue mixing for another 2-3 minutes. Spoon into a pastry bag with cake decorating tip and pipe on top of cupcakes.

Store cupcakes at room temperature for up to 3 days, or in freezer for up to 6 months.

Chocolate Ice Cream ⚱ (1 quart)

2 ¾ cups heavy whipping cream, divided
1 cup chocolate chips

14 oz. can sweetened condensed milk
1 tbsp. vanilla extract

Heat ½ cup heavy cream in a microwave safe dish for 30-45 seconds, or until it starts to boil. Pour over chocolate chips in a small mixing bowl and whisk together well until chocolate is melted and smooth, set aside. In a large mixing bowl, whisk together sweetened condensed milk and vanilla. Add melted chocolate and whisk again until well combined, set aside. In a standing mixer or another medium size mixing bowl, beat 2 ¼ cups heavy cream at high speed until stiff peaks form. Spoon half of whipped cream into chocolate mixture, stir together with a spatula until well combined. Add remaining whipped cream and repeat process. Pour into a bowl, loaf pan, or quart container. Cover and place in freezer for a minimum of 4 hours to set.

Chocolate Mousse ⚱ (4-6 servings)

½ cup + 2/3 cup heavy whipping cream
1 cup chocolate chips

1 tbsp. confectioners sugar
Whipped Cream (p. 214)

Heat ½ cup heavy cream in a microwave safe dish for 30-45 seconds until bubbling, pour over chocolate chips in a small mixing bowl. Whisk together well until chocolate is melted and smooth, set aside to cool to room temperature (about 15 minutes). Beat 2/3 cup heavy cream in a medium size mixing bowl with confectioners sugar until stiff peaks form. When chocolate has cooled to room temperature, fold the whipped cream into melted chocolate until fully combined. Transfer to individual dishes and chill for at least 2 hours before serving. Top with Whipped Cream when ready to serve.

Chocolate Peanut Butter Bars ⚱ (12-16 servings)

½ cup butter, softened
1 ¾ cup confectioners sugar
1 cup creamy peanut butter

¾ cup gluten-free graham cracker crumbs
1 cup semisweet chocolate chips
½ cup heavy cream

Line a square 8x8 inch pan with foil, leaving enough to hang over sides. Rub a little bit of butter on bottom and sides to help prevent the bars from sticking. In a medium saucepan, melt ½ cup butter over low heat. Once melted, remove from heat and stir in confectioners sugar until smooth. Add peanut butter and graham cracker crumbs, stir until completely combined and smooth. Spread the mixture into the pan in an even layer. Heat heavy cream in a microwave safe dish for 45-60 seconds, just until it starts to bubble. Pour over chocolate chips in a small mixing bowl and whisk together well until chocolate is melted and smooth. Spread chocolate over peanut butter layer and place pan in refrigerator to set for at least 30 minutes. Remove from pan using the foil overhangs and place on a cutting board to slice into bars. Store in airtight container in refrigerator for up to 1 week.

Crème Brulee ♨ *(6-8 servings)*

1 whole egg
4 egg yolks
½ cup granulated sugar

3 cups heavy cream
1 tbsp. triple sec
2 tsp. vanilla extract

Preheat oven to 300 degrees. Whisk together the egg, yolks, and sugar in a medium size mixing bowl, set aside. In a microwave safe container, heat the heat creamy until hot but not quite boiling. Slowly pour a stream of the cream into the bowl with the egg mixture, constantly whisking. Add the triple sec and vanilla, whisk again. Pour liquid through a wire mesh strainer into another bowl with a spout. Pour into 6-8 shallow ramekins. Place in a half sheet cake pan and pour hot water into pan surrounding the ramekins (be careful not to get water into ramekins). Carefully place pan in the oven and bake for 40-50 minutes, just until the custards are set and just a tiny bit jiggly. Remove pan from oven, use spatula to transfer ramekins to a cooling rack. When they have cooled completely, cover with plastic wrap and store in refrigerator for at least 4 hours before serving. When ready to serve, sprinkle 1-2 teaspoons granulated sugar evenly on top of custard and torch the top using a kitchen torch. Let set for 1 minute before serving.

Pro-Tip: for **Chocolate Crème Brulee**: add 8 oz. chopped bittersweet chocolate to heavy cream before heating in microwave, whisk until melted before adding to yolk mixture. Replace triple sec with ¼ cup coffee liquor. You're welcome.

Dinner Rolls ♨ *(16 servings)*

3 ¼ cups gluten-free all-purpose flour
1 cup tapioca starch, divided
4 tsp. instant yeast
¼ cup granulated sugar

1 tsp. sea salt
13 oz. warm milk (90 degrees)
½ cup butter, melted
2 egg whites (room temperature)

In the bowl of a standing mixer, combine flour, 7/8 cup tapioca starch, yeast, granulated sugar, and salt, whisk together well. Add milk, butter, egg whites, and beat vigorously using the paddle attachment. It will come together in a clump and clear the sides of the bowl. Continue beating until it starts to look whipped and sticks to the side of the mixing bowl, which takes about 6 minutes. Transfer dough to a lightly oiled large bowl and cover tightly with plastic wrap. Set aside for at least 2 hours at room temperature. Coat a quarter sheet pan with cooking spray and set aside. Divide dough into 16 equal portions, about 2.5 oz. in weight. One piece at a time, knead dough using clean, dry hands and pinch any seams that separate. Sprinkle a dry work surface with remaining tapioca starch and form them into balls. Arrange in baking sheet and cover with lightly greased plastic wrap, place in a warm location and allow to rise about 150% their original size. This process can take at least 45 minutes, depending on the temperature in your kitchen. When rolls are almost done rising, preheat oven to 375 degrees. When rolls are ready, brush with melted butter. Place pan in oven to bake for 18-20 minutes, or until internal thermometer reads 190 degrees. Serve warm.

Fathead Dough ♟ (4-6 servings)

2 ½ cups grated mozzarella cheese
2 oz. cream cheese, softened
2 eggs

2 tbsp. baking powder
½ tsp. onion powder
3 cups almond flour

Melt cheese in microwave for 3 minutes, stir and melt an additional minute if needed. Transfer to a standing mixer, add eggs, then baking powder, onion powder, and almond flour. Use dough hook and mix at medium speed until completely incorporated and forms into dough. Use as needed for a variety of recipes or wrap dough in plastic wrap and refrigerate for 24 hours until ready to use.

Pro-Tip: this is a base recipe for low carb/keto dough and can be used to make pizzas, bagels, dinner rolls, breadsticks, and more! You can also add Italian seasoning and garlic powder for more flavor and use sharp cheddar cheese to make cheesy rolls.

Garlic Breadsticks ♟♟ (12 servings)

4 ¼ cups gluten-free all-purpose flour
2 tsp. instant yeast
2 tbsp. granulated sugar
2 tsp. sea salt

6 tbsp. butter, softened
11 oz. warm water (90 degrees)
3 tbsp. butter, melted
1 tsp. garlic salt

In the bowl of a standing mixer, combine flour, yeast, granulated sugar, and salt, whisk together well. Add softened butter and warm water, mix on low speed with dough hook until combined. Increase mixer speed to medium and knead for about five minutes, until dough is sticky but should be smooth and stretchy. Grease a silicone spatula with cooking spray, scrape down the sides of the bowl. Line a rimmed baking sheet with parchment paper and set aside. Sprinkle a clean work surface with extra flour and knead with your hands until smooth. Divide into 12 equal pieces, about 3.5 oz. each. Working with one piece at a time, shape into a rectangle that is about ½ inch thick and 4 inches long. Fold rectangle halfway along the length from bottom to top, then top to bottom. Roll the dough back and forth gently on a lightly floured surface to seal the edges well, elongated until the dough is about 7 inches long with tapered dough on both ends. Place each piece on the prepared baking sheet, about 2 inches apart from each other. When all breadsticks are shaped, cover baking sheet with greased plastic wrap and place in a warm place to rise until the breadsticks are almost doubled in size, which will take about 1 hour. About 20 minutes before dough has finished rising, preheat oven to 375 degrees and remove plastic wrap. Place baking sheet in oven and immediately decrease temperature to 350 degrees, bake for 5 minutes. While bread is baking, melt butter in a small microwave safe dish or saucepan. Add garlic salt and whisk together. Remove baking sheet from oven, brush with garlic butter and place sheet back in oven to bake for another 5 minutes. Remove from oven and brush with more garlic butter, serve warm.

M&M® Brownies ⚱ *(12-24 servings)*

2 boxes gluten-free brownie mix
1 cup vegetable oil
4 eggs

¼ cup water
10 oz. bag mini M&Ms®

Preheat oven to 350 degrees. Line a 9x13 inch baking pan with parchment paper hanging over sides, coat with cooking spray. Dump both bags of brownie mixes into a large mixing bowl. Combine oil, eggs, and water in a small mixing bowl and whisk together well. Pour liquid into large mixing bowl with brownie mixes and stir together gently with a spatula until well-combined. Spoon batter into pan on top of parchment paper and spread into an even layer. Sprinkle bag of M&Ms® on top of batter. Place pan in oven and bake for about 50 minutes, until a toothpick inserted in center comes out with just a tiny bit of fudge on tip. Set pan on cooling rack to cool completely. Remove brownies from pan by pulling up sides of parchment paper and transfer to a cutting board. Cut brownies into desired sizes and store in airtight container for 3 days or wrap individually and store in the freezer for up to 6 months.

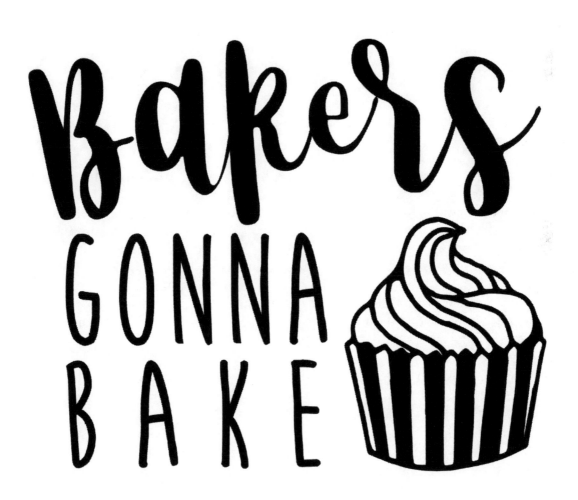

Bakers Gonna Bake

New York Cheesecake 🍴 *(8-12 servings)*

For the Crust
1 ¼ cups gluten-free graham cracker crumbs
2 tbsp. granulated sugar
5 tbsp. butter, melted

For the Toppings
Whipped Cream

For The Filling
4 (8 oz.) packages cream cheese, softened
¼ cup cornstarch
1 2/3 cups granulated sugar
2 eggs
1 tbsp. vanilla extract
¾ cup heavy cream

Preheat oven to 350 degrees. Double wrap the outside of a 9-inch springform pan with heavy duty aluminum foil, place inside a 12-inch cake pan. Place graham cracker crumbs and 2 tablespoons sugar in a small mixing bowl, toss together. Add the melted butter and mix with your hands or a spatula until thoroughly combined. Grease the bottom of the springform pan with cooking spray, then press graham cracker mixture evenly along the bottom. Place pans in the oven to bake for 7 minutes, remove pans from oven and set aside.

In a standing mixer, combine 8 oz. cream cheese, cornstarch, and 2/3 cups sugar. Beat at medium speed with the paddle attachment until mixture is smooth. Add another 8 oz. cream cheese, along with 1/3 cup sugar and continue to beat until smooth. Add remaining cream cheese and granulated sugar, one at a time, beat until smooth. Slow mixer to stirring speed, add vanilla and one egg at a time, scraping down the sides. Turn on to stirring speed and slowly add heavy cream just until mixed in (do not overmix). Spoon mixture into springform pan on top of graham cracker crust and spread into an even layer.

Pour warm water into the larger cake pan, creating a water bath (this helps prevent cracks). The water should come up about 1 inch around the springform pan. Carefully place pans in oven and bake for about 1 hour 15 minutes, until lightly browned on top. Remove pans from oven, pull the springform pan out of the larger pan and place on a cooling rack for about 4 hours to cool completely. Remove aluminum foil from around pan. Cover springform pan with plastic wrap and place in freezer to set for at least 4 hours; preferably overnight. Remove plastic wrap from springform pan. Release and remove sides of springform. Place a piece of parchment or wax paper on top of cheesecake, turn upside down on a flat surface. Carefully remove bottom of pan using a sharp knife, turn back over onto a serving plate.

Cut into slices with a sharp, straight edged knife, wiping knife between each cut. Store cheesecake in refrigerator until ready to serve for up to 5 days, or in the freezer for 1 month. Serve with whipped cream, Strawberry Sauce (p. 90), or other toppings as desired.

Pro-Tip: as a whole, cheesecakes can easily be made gluten-free just by making sure the crust and toppings don't contain gluten since the filling doesn't have it. Feel free to experiment with different flavors, fillings, and toppings to your heart's desire.

Oreo® Trifle (10-12 servings)

1 box gluten-free brownie mix
1 package gluten-free Oreo® cookies
2 small boxes instant chocolate pudding mix

4 cups milk, divided
8 oz. frozen whipped topping, thawed

Following directions on brownie box, bake brownies in oven in a 9x13 inch baking dish and cool completely. Combine pudding mix and 3 cups milk in a medium size mixing bowl, whisk until blended. Take half of brownies and crumble into bottom of a trifle bowl. Spoon half of pudding mixture on top of brownies. Dip half of cookies in remaining milk (to soften) and place on top of pudding mixture in bowl. Spoon half of remaining whipped topping on top of Oreo® layer. Repeat layering. Garnish with an extra crumbled cookie if desired, top with a piece of plastic wrap and store in refrigerator for at least 2 hours before serving.

Oreo® Truffles (40-50 truffles)

1 package gluten-free Oreo® cookies
8 oz. cream cheese, softened

2 (10 oz.) bags dark chocolate melting wafers
2-4 oz. white chocolate melting wafers

Using a food processor, grind cookies into fine crumbs. Combine crumbs with cream cheese in a medium size mixing bowl and beat with electric mixer at medium speed until well blended. Using a mini-ice cream scoop, spoon out portions onto a cookie sheet lined with wax paper. Transfer to refrigerator to set for about 1 hour. Melt dark chocolate in a microwave safe dish in 30 second intervals, stirring after each time until chocolate is completely melted. Be careful not to overheat, the chocolate will scald and clump together! Pull the truffle balls out of the fridge, re-roll with hands for a smooth consistency. Using a toothpick, insert into each ball, dip into melted dark chocolate to fully cover, gently shake off excess chocolate and place back on wax paper. Return to refrigerator for chocolate to set, melt white chocolate and drizzle on top. Transfer each truffle to a mini muffin liner for easy serving, store in refrigerator until ready to serve.

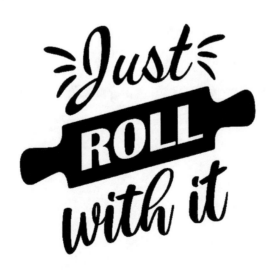

Peanut Butter Cup Ice Cream *(1 quart)*

14 oz. can sweetened condensed milk
¾ cup creamy peanut butter
1 tbsp. vanilla

2 ¼ cups heavy cream, divided
4 peanut butter cups, chopped

Combine sweetened condensed milk, peanut butter, vanilla, and ¼ cup heavy cream in a blender and puree until smooth. Pour peanut butter mixture into a large mixing bowl. In a standing mixer or medium size mixing bowl, beat the remaining 2 cups heavy cream at high speed until stiff peaks form. Spoon half of whipped cream into peanut butter mixture, stir together with a spatula until well combined. Add remaining whipped cream and repeat process. Add chopped peanut butter cups and stir. Pour into a bowl, loaf pan, or quart container. Cover and place in freezer for a minimum of 4 hours to set before serving.

Pro-Tip: for even more chocolate, drizzle some chocolate syrup on top of the ice cream after you have scooped it into the container, or just save it for serving. Remember to check ingredients to make sure your chocolate syrup is gluten-free!

Pie Crust *(2 pie crusts)*

1 ½ cups gluten-free all-purpose flour
1/3 cup confectioners sugar
¼ tsp. sea salt
9 tbsp. butter

½ tsp. vanilla extract
1 egg yolk
3 tbsp. ice cold water

Cut butter into small chunks, place in a small mixing bowl and place in refrigerator. In a large mixing bowl or food processor, whisk together the flour, sugar, and salt. Add cold butter. Use a pastry tool (or pulse if using a food processor), cut butter into flour mixture until it resembles a coarse meal. In a small bowl, whisk together yolks, ice cold water, and vanilla until combined. Add to flour mixture, tossing with a fork or pulsing until incorporated. Form dough into a ball and divide into 2 pieces. Form each piece into a ball and flatten to form disks. Wrap each disk separately in plastic wrap, chill for at least 1 hour and up to 1 week in refrigerator, or up to 1 month in freezer. Use as needed in recipes.

Pro-Tip: for a **Savory Pie Crust**, omit confectioners sugar.

Pizza Dough (1 crust)

2 cups gluten-free all-purpose flour
1 tbsp. baking powder
1 tsp. salt

1 tsp. Italian seasoning
2 tbsp. olive oil
¾ cup warm water

Preheat oven to 375 degrees. Combine all ingredients in a medium size mixing bowl or standing mixer, beat at medium speed with electric mixer until well-combined. Add extra water as needed if the dough is too thick. Form dough into a ball, brush a little extra olive oil on top and place in refrigerator for at least 10 minutes. Place cold dough on a piece of parchment paper, place another piece of parchment paper on top of the dough. Using a rolling pin, roll into a large circle (about 10-12 inches in diameter). Transfer dough to a pizza stone or baking sheet, poke holes in crust using a fork. Place pan in oven and bake for 10-12 minutes, until golden. Remove crust from oven, top with sauce, cheese, and toppings. Bake for another 8-10 minutes or until cheese is melted.

Pro-Tip: this is a very simple recipe for pizza dough, so if you want a dough that's make-your-knees-buckle amazing, feel free to do some searching for other highly rated recipes using yeast. I decided to choose a simple recipe for this book because many people are looking for something quick and easy to throw together for pizza night. Well, mainly it's me looking for something a little easier for pizza night. Guilty as charged.

Pound Cake (8-10 servings)

1 lb. butter, softened
1 cup granulated sugar
5 eggs
1 tsp. vanilla extract

1 tsp. almond extract
1 2/3 cups gluten-free all-purpose flour
1 tsp. sea salt

Preheat oven to 325 degrees. Grease a 9x5 inch loaf pan and set aside. Place butter in a medium size mixing bowl or standing mixer with paddle attachment, beat at medium-high speed until light and fluffy. Slowly add sugar, eggs, and extracts, while mixer is on low speed, then increase speed and beat until smooth. In another small mixing bowl, whisk together flour and salt. Add the flour mixture (about ¼ cup at a time), mixing just until combined. The batter will be thick, but smooth. Spoon mixture into loaf pan and smooth top with a wet spatula. Place pan in oven and bake for about 50 minutes, rotating once during baking time. When cake is lightly golden brown all over and a toothpick inserted in the center comes out clean, remove pan from oven. Place on cooling rack and cool in pan for at least 30 minutes before removing from the pan and allow to cool completely. Slice into 1 inch thick pieces, store in airtight container at room temperature for up to 3 days or wrap individually in plastic wrap and store in freezer for up to 6 months.

Pumpkin Bread 🍴 *(2 loaves)*

2 cups gluten-free all-purpose flour
½ tsp. salt
1 tsp. baking soda
½ tsp. baking powder
2 tsp. ground cinnamon
1 tsp. ground nutmeg

¾ cup butter, softened
1 cup granulated sugar
1 cup light brown sugar
2 large eggs
15 oz. can pureed pumpkin

Preheat oven to 325 degrees. Grease two 4x8 inch loaf pans with cooking spray and lightly sprinkle with extra gluten-free all-purpose flour, set aside. In a medium size mixing bowl, combine flour, salt, baking soda, baking powder, cinnamon, and nutmeg. Whisk until combined, set aside. In a large mixing bowl, beat butter and sugars at medium speed just until blended. Add eggs one at a time, beating well after each addition. Continue mixing until light and fluffy, about 2 minutes. Add pumpkin and beat again. Add flour mixture and mix on low speed until combined. Spoon batter evenly into prepared pans, place pans in oven and bake for 50-55 minutes or until a toothpick inserted in the center comes out clean. Place pans on cooling racks and cool for about 10 minutes before turning loaves out of pans to cool completely on cooling racks.

🍴 **Pro-Tip:** to change your life for the better, smother this bread with Cinnamon Honey Butter: just add ½ tsp. ground cinnamon to the Honey Butter recipe (p. 27).

Pumpkin Oatmeal Cookies 🍴🍴 *(3-4 dozen cookies)*

1 ½ cups butter, softened
2 cups light brown sugar
1 cup granulated sugar
2 tbsp. molasses
15 oz. can pureed pumpkin
1 egg
1 tbsp. vanilla
4 cups gluten-free all-purpose flour

2 tsp. cinnamon
2 tsp. baking soda
1 tsp. baking powder
1 tsp. salt
6 cups old fashioned oats
1 cup confectioners sugar
2-3 tbsp. milk or water

Preheat oven to 375 degrees. Combine butter and sugars in a large mixing bowl and beat at medium speed with electric mixer until light and fluffy, about 2 minutes. Add molasses, pumpkin, egg, and vanilla, continue beating for another 30 seconds. Add flour, cinnamon, baking soda, baking powder, and salt, continue mixing again. Add oats and beat just until combined. Using a cookie scoop, distribute dough to silicone or parchment lined baking sheets, gently press down and bake for 11-12 minutes. Remove pan from oven, let cookies sit on pan for 2-3 minutes before transferring to cooling racks to cool completely. In a small bowl, combine confectioners sugar and milk, drizzle on top of cookies. Store cookies in airtight container at room temperature for up to 5 days or wrap individually with plastic wrap and store in freezer for up to 6 months.

Sandwich Bread 🍴 *(1 loaf)*

3 cups gluten-free all-purpose flour
2 ½ tsp. gluten-free instant yeast
¼ tsp. cream of tartar
2 tbsp. granulated sugar
2 tsp. salt

1 ½ cups milk (about 90 degrees)
¼ cup butter, melted
1 tsp. apple cider vinegar
2 egg whites at room temperature
¼ tsp. vanilla

Grease a 9x5 inch loaf pan with cooking spray, or line it with parchment paper and set aside. In a standing mixer, combine flour, yeast, cream of tartar, sugar, and salt, whisk to combine. Add milk, butter, apple cider vinegar, egg whites, and vanilla, mixing on low speed with the paddle attachment after each addition. Scrape down the sides of the bowl with a spatula as needed while mixing. Mix at medium speed for about 3 minutes, the dough will be thick. Transfer dough to loaf pan and use a wet spatula to smooth the top. Cover with plastic wrap that has been lightly oiled, allow dough to rise in a warm place for about 45 minutes or until it's about 150% larger than its original size. Preheat oven to 375 degrees. Remove plastic wrap and use a sharp knife to cut a long slit about ¼ inch deep in the dough. Brush with more melted butter, if desired. Bake in oven for 45-60 minutes, or until internal thermometer reads 195 degrees and bread has a thick, brown crust. Remove pan from oven, cool in pan for 10 minutes then transfer to cooling rack to cool completely. Slice and wrap each piece individually in plastic wrap, use within 3 days or store in freezer for up to 6 months.

Pro-Tip: Better Batter® brand was used in this recipe and does contain xanthan gum. If flour does not already contain xanthan gum, add 2 ¼ tsp. to the recipe.

Snickerdoodles 🍴 *(2 dozen)*

1 cup oat flour
1 ¾ cups gluten-free all-purpose flour
1 tsp. baking powder
1 tsp. baking soda
1 tsp. sea salt
1 tsp. cinnamon
1 cup butter, softened

1 cup light brown sugar
1 cup granulated sugar
1 tbsp. honey
2 eggs
2 tsp. vanilla
¼ cup granulated cinnamon
1 tbsp. cinnamon

Preheat oven to 350 degrees. In a small mixing bowl, combine flours, baking powder, baking soda, salt, cinnamon, whisk together and set aside. Combine softened butter and sugars in a medium size mixing bowl and beat at medium speed with electric mixer until light and fluffy. Add honey, eggs, and vanilla, continue mixing just until combined. Add dry ingredients in two batches, beat in between each to incorporate well. Using a cookie scoop, drop dough on silicone lined cookie sheet. Stir together the remaining cinnamon and sugar, lightly press each cookie in mixture and place on cookie sheet. Bake for approximately 12 minutes or until lightly golden. Let cookies sit on cookie sheet for another 2-3 minutes before transferring to cooling racks.

Strawberry Shortcakes ♀ *(12 servings)*

2 1/3 cups gluten-free Bisquick
¼ cup granulated sugar
¼ cup butter, melted

½ cup milk
Strawberry Sauce (pg. 90)
Whipped Cream (p. 214)

Preheat oven to 425 degrees. In a medium size mixing bowl, combine all ingredients and stir until a soft dough forms. Drop dough on a silicone lined baking sheet using a cookie scoop, then slightly push down on each biscuit. Place pan in oven and bake for 10-12 minutes, or until lightly golden. Cool slightly and slice each biscuit in half, place bottom on a plate. Top with strawberry sauce, other shortcake half, more sauce, and garnish with whipped cream.

Vanilla Cupcakes ♀ *(24 cupcakes)*

For the Cupcakes

1 box gluten-free yellow cake mix*
1 small box Jell-O® instant vanilla pudding mix
¾ cup vegetable oil

½ cup milk
4 eggs
8 oz. sour cream

Preheat oven to 350 degrees. Combine all ingredients in a medium size mixing bowl or standing mixer, beat at medium speed for 1-2 minutes until batter is smooth. Scoop batter into lined muffin pans, place in oven to bake for 21-23 minutes, until a toothpick inserted in center of cupcakes comes out clean. Remove pans from oven, remove cupcakes from pans to cool completely on cooling racks.

*The gluten-free cake mix used in this recipe is King Arthur® brand. These measurements are based on recipe experiments using this brand. If you use another brand and something comes off wonky, you've been warned. Love you, mean it.

For Vanilla Buttercream Icing

1 lb. butter, softened
6 cups confectioners sugar
1 tbsp. vanilla extract
¼ cup milk
Colorful sprinkles

For Pink Almond Icing

1 lb. butter, softened
6 cups confectioners sugar
1 tsp. almond extract
¼ cup milk
1 tsp. pink food coloring

Beat butter at high speed in a medium size mixing bowl or standing mixer for at least 3 minutes, until light and fluffy. Add remaining ingredients and beat slowly to incorporate, then increase speed to high and continue mixing for another 2-3 minutes. Spoon into a pastry bag with cake decorating tip and pipe on top of cupcakes. Garnish with sprinkles, if desired.

Vanilla Ice Cream ⚲ *(1 quart)*

14 oz. can sweetened condensed milk   2 cups heavy cream
1 tbsp. vanilla

Combine sweetened condensed milk and vanilla in a large mixing bowl and whisk together well, set aside. In a standing mixer or medium size mixing bowl, beat the heavy cream at high speed until stiff peaks form. Spoon half of whipped cream into condensed milk and vanilla mixture, stir together with a spatula until well combined. Add remaining whipped cream and repeat process. Pour into a bowl, loaf pan, or quart container and add any extras you prefer. Cover and place in freezer for a minimum of 4 hours to set.

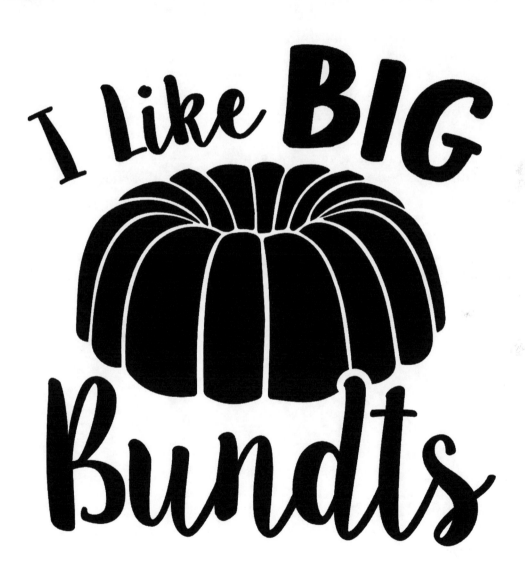

Specialty Diet Recipe Index

Since there are so many diets for different individuals, the recipes have been categorized into types of diets. Feel free to grab different colored highlighters or sticky notes and go to town if you're looking for specialty recipes...but only if this is your book, of course.

Traditional- traditional recipes that have absolutely no limitations and include everything under the sun...except gluten, of course. That would derail the purpose of this book, and we don't want to do that.

Blue Zones (Mediterranean)- recipes that focus on mostly whole foods with minimal dairy and processed foods, but do contain beans, grains, meat, and eggs.

Dairy-Free- recipes that do not contain any dairy, *or* recipes that can be converted easily into dairy-free simply by using dairy-free butter and/or dairy-free milk.

Low-Carb- recipes that do not contain foods with higher amounts of carbs, such as rice, potatoes, oats, flour, grains, beans, etc.

Plant-Based- recipes that do not contain any meat, eggs, dairy, or processed sugar. They do contain sweeteners such as honey, maple syrup, and stevia.

Vegan- recipes that do not have any animal products; meat, eggs, dairy, honey, but do contain all other forms of sugar.

Vegetarian- recipes that do not contain meat but do contain eggs and/or dairy.

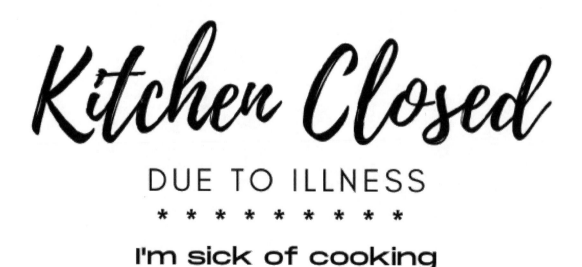

Traditional (all recipes)

Blue Zones (Mediterranean)

What are Blue Zones?

Blue Zones are the five regions of the world where people live the longest and are said to be the healthiest, where many of them consistently reach the age of 100. They are less likely to suffer from chronic illnesses, stay active, prioritize stress relief, eat a largely plant-based diet (but overall, more of a Mediterranean Style Diet), drink alcohol in moderation, and have healthy social relationships. There are multiple books and documentaries on these regions and the lifestyles people live, and it's quite different and fascinating from most of the overly developed areas of the world.

The Five Blue Zones are:
1. Sardinia, Italy
2. Okinawa, Japan
3. Loma Linda, California
4. Ikaria, Greece
5. Nicoya, Costa Rica

Dairy-Free

Low-Carb

What is the difference between Keto and Paleo?

Although both Keto and Paleo Diets are considered Low-Carb, there are differences
between them. Keto focuses on extremely low-carb, high fat, dairy, only a small number
of low-carb fruits (like berries), and sweeteners such as erythritol and monkfruit. Paleo
is considered *lower* carb but not as low as Keto, has no limitations on fruits, allows
smaller amounts of sugar from maple syrup and honey, and no dairy consumption.

Plant-Based

Vegan

Vegetarian

Thank you so much for purchasing this book! I sincerely hope it becomes your new favorite kitchen necessity and opens the flood gates for incredible meals for you to enjoy with your friends and family. If you can spare the time, I would greatly appreciate it if you could leave a review on Amazon and share your experience with this book. Thanks again and stay tuned for many more books in the future!!

Interested in buying 10 or more copies? Please contact us for discount prices!

E-mail: ekirk713@gmail.com

Check out...

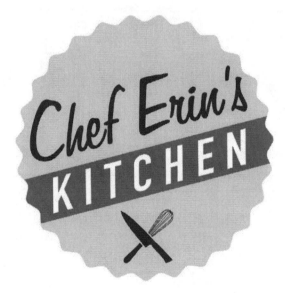

on YouTube, Facebook, and Instagram!

For recipe videos, pictures, and lots of dorky humor. You've been warned.

www.cheferinskitchen.com

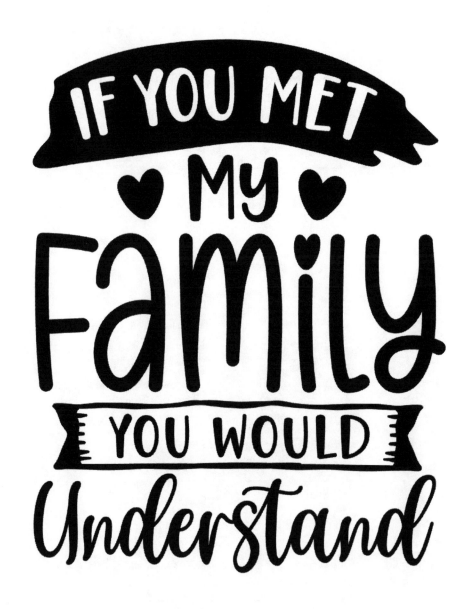

Made in United States
Orlando, FL
05 October 2023

37616959R00135